Discoveries in Biological Psychiatry

SECOND ANNUAL TAYLOR MANOR HOSPITAL SCIENTIFIC SYMPOSIUM

DISCOVERIES IN BIOLOGICAL PSYCHIATRY

BALTIMORE MARYLAND APRIL 1970

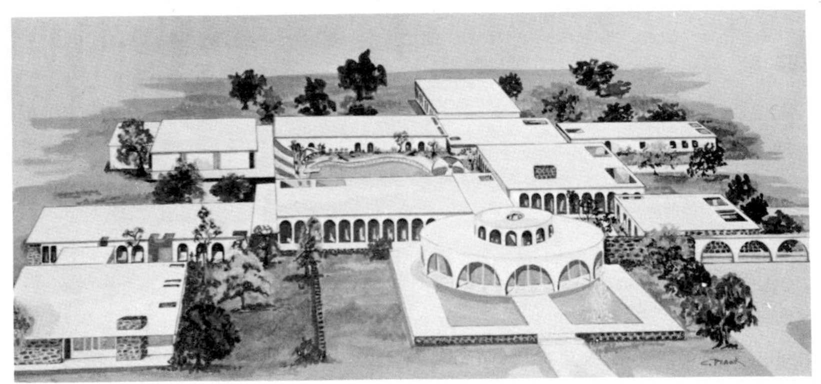

Taylor Manor Hospital, Ellicott City, Maryland

Discoveries in Biological Psychiatry

Edited by

Frank J. Ayd, Jr., MD, FAPA

Editor: *International Drug Therapy Newsletter*
Medical-Moral Newsletter

and

Barry Blackwell, MD, DPM

Associate Professor of Psychiatry and Pharmacology, University of Cincinnati, Group Director, Psychiatric Clinical Research, The Wm. S. Merrell Company, Cincinnati

J. B. LIPPINCOTT COMPANY

Philadelphia/Toronto

Distributed in Great Britain by
Blackwell Scientific Publications
Oxford and Edinburgh

Library of Congress Catalog Card No. 78-124542

PRINTED IN THE UNITED STATES OF AMERICA
SP-B

Dedicated to
Dr. and Mrs. Irving J. Taylor
and to
our wives

Preface

THIS BOOK SHARES the same purpose as the symposium from which its contents are derived. Gathered here are the accounts of all the original discoveries in biological psychiatry, recounted, as far as possible, by those who made them. In addition to the enjoyment and vicarious excitement of these reports, the book serves a threefold purpose: as a historical record, a teaching instrument, and an encouragement to other clinicians and research workers.

Never previously has an attempt been made to gather these accounts together and, in some instances, the tales are related publically for the first time. It is an index of the remarkable speed of progress in this area that so many of the accounts could be rendered by the authors themselves while still within easy recollection. These eminent scientists and clinicians were asked to tell the story of their discovery in their own personal manner. Not surprisingly, they have chosen to do so in different ways, with varying emphases on one or another aspect of the process of discovery. Rather than editorially confining the accounts within an artificial format, we have deliberately chosen to allow the author complete freedom. Some have plunged straight into a personal and intimate account, while others have eschewed this viewpoint to emphasize the purely scientific aspects. Several contributors preferred to fit their discovery into the pattern of a lifework; others have adhered strictly to an individual episode.

There are as many ways of describing a discovery as there are of making it, but the discerning reader should have no problem in appreciating the lessons he may learn from each of these accounts.

The sheer pace of these innovations as well as their number has created problems for those whose task it is to teach physical methods of treatment in psychiatry to medical or pharmacy students and psychiatric residents, as well as to the host of paramedical workers who assist in applying the tools of biological psychiatry to implement community care. In talking to such diverse audiences, one finds that historical perspective aids understanding, provides a rational framework, and imparts additional interest.

Compared to the fruitful years recorded here, biological psychiatry has fallen on more barren times. It is not unusual for an era of productivity to be followed by the kind of slack interval in which we are currently becalmed. If nothing else, such moments provide a time for reminiscence from which it is possible to draw fresh momentum. There is a simplicity about accounts of discovery that somehow encourages the belief that one day it might happen to us. It probably can. For even in an era of research sophistication, we may recall Charles Darwin's wry observation: "I love fool's experiments, I am always making them." Whether the readers of this book are research workers or busy clinicians, these reports by others like them illustrate how close observation and continual questioning may lead not only to original discoveries but also to better medicine.

THE EDITORS

Contents

CHAPTER

1

The Process of Discovery

Barry Blackwell, MD, DPM *

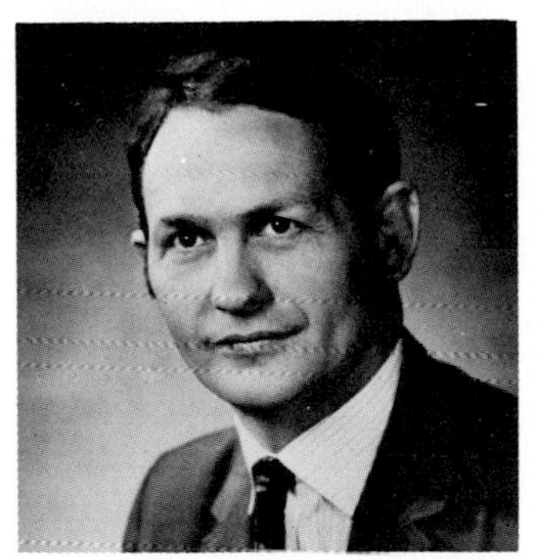

The intention of this meeting can be simply stated: to garner a personal record of outstanding discoveries in biological psychiatry and to commend those who made them. At a moment when the pace of discovery has slackened, it is possible that further advances may be stimulated by a timely backward glance. William Mayo put this succinctly in his remarks on the romance of medicine: "It is a great thing to make scientific discoveries of rare value, but it is even greater to be willing to share these discoveries and to encourage other workers in the same field of scientific research." [1]

A personal fascination with this theme sprang from sharing in the discovery of an unwelcome side effect rather than the finding of a new drug. This was the hypertensive crisis provoked by cheese in patients prescribed monoamine oxidase inhibitors.[2] Later on, the preparation of lectures in psychopharmacology for residents revealed only scanty accounts of the more important discoveries in biological psychiatry and nurtured a wish to see them adequately documented and gathered together while still within easy recollection. It was during a mutual discussion of this need with Dr. Frank Ayd last year that the seeds of this meeting took root.

Until the preparation of this paper, I had naively assumed that intimate accounts of the discovery process in other areas were

* Associate Professor of Psychiatry and Pharmacology, University of Cincinnati, Group Director, Psychiatric Clinical Research, The Wm. S. Merrell Company, Cincinnati.

equally rare and limited to celebrated examples like Newton's apple and Archimedes bath.[3] Instead, there exist a plethora of detailed reports. For instance, Lipetz's *A Guide to Case Studies of Scientific Activity*[4] provides an annotated bibliography of over 300 such accounts, the majority published in the last 20 years and ranging from the more classical discoveries of Nobel Prize winners to mundane sagas of invention which include the electric light, nylon, and even the problems in development of clam farms. More detailed accounts of over 50 outstanding discoveries are set forth in Garrett's *The Flash of Genius*,[5] and there are many books devoted to individual discoveries, several of which have become popular best sellers.[6-12] Quite apart from these descriptions of discovery themselves, there have been many examinations of the processes involved[3, 10, 13-32] and the psychological attributes of the scientists concerned including their intellectual, motivational, and personality characteristics.[33-43] The whole topic of the scientists' behavior in the discovery process has become almost a subspecialty of sociological inquiry, in which Robert Merton's detailed reviews make both fascinating and chastening reading.[44-48]

Rather than attempt to summarize this wealth of material, I have chosen to dissect a personal discovery and, by analogy with other more important findings, to anticipate some of the common threads that will run through the accounts ahead.

BEGINNINGS OF DISCOVERY

The story of how a discovery began may be as instructive as the way in which it was exploited, yet research workers are usually reticent about the clues that initiate an investigation. The first steps are often forgotten in the excitement of continuing discovery, so that what appears in retrospect to be a process of brilliant inductive reasoning began, in fact, as a series of blindfold leaps in the dark. This reticence serves the dual purpose of preserving scientific self-esteem and conforming with research etiquette. Unfortunately, it is also more likely to stifle the fair allocation of credit than to conceal modesty. Robert Merton[48] has illustrated this process of "vast expurgation" by contrasting the 900 words of Crick and Watson's historic article in *Nature* describing the double helix with the "tangled web of events" reported in Watson's later 40,000 word account of the same discovery.[9]

In looking back over the story of the cheese reaction, the same process of abbreviation becomes apparent. As an intern in neurology, I worked under a resident who had previously published an account of subarachnoid hemorrhage in a patient taking a monoamine oxidase inhibitor.[49] For this reason, I learned to take a drug history in all such cases. The search remained unrewarded, but during the next appointment as a junior resident in psychiatry at the Maudsley Hospital, I heard of a similar incident in a patient who was taking tranylcypromine. During the preceding 20 months, there had been 6 independent reports of such cases in letters to the *Lancet*.[50-55] A discussion with a local general practitioner revealed that he was unpleasantly familiar with the syndrome and had been called from his bed twice within a week to see patients taking monoamine oxidase inhibitors who complained of sudden severe headache.

These coincidences impelled me to write a letter to the *Lancet* drawing attention to the fairly frequent association of hypertension and a picture resembling or even causing subarachnoid hemorrhage in patients taking monoamine oxidase inhibitors.[56] That letter had important sequels. A hospital pharmacist in Nottingham (G. E. F. Rowe) read the *Lancet* and recognized the symptoms as identical to those his wife had experienced twice after eating cheese. He described the episodes in detail in a letter that concluded:

> Could there be a link between the effects and the amino acids of the cheese? No effects are caused by butter or milk. Although treatment has continued, no further episodes have occurred. If cheese is indeed the factor, it could perhaps explain the sporadic nature of the incidence of the side effect. I hope my comments will be of some use to you in your investigations. (G. E. F. Rowe)

The letter was shown to several colleagues who shared my amusement before I then wrote a brief reply dismissing the notion. But not everyone was so skeptical. Later that same week, a drug salesman (Mr. Gerald Samuel), with whom this incident was also shared, recalled two similar reports the pharmaceutical company had received but dismissed. He had also heard of a death the previous week in another hospital he called on, which occurred during treatment with an MAOI and an amino acid. The encouragement and stimulus were now sufficient to arouse action. Consultation of the hospital diet sheets revealed that on the night of the incident the Maudsley patient (who was a vegetarian) had eaten a cheese pie.

The next and obvious step was an attempt to provoke the reaction experimentally. A colleague and I took tranylcypromine for a week and then sat down to a breakfast of cheese; nothing happened. This was a discouraging moment, not least because of the gathering ridicule that the "cheese idea" was attracting among fellow residents. The disappointment might have stifled further inquiry but for another coincidence. During a weekend on duty for a local general practitioner, a call came to visit a patient suffering from sudden severe headache; she was taking phenelzine, had eaten cheese sandwiches for supper, and was in the midst of a hypertensive crisis.

It now seemed inevitable that another attempt be made to induce the condition experimentally. A volunteer patient taking tranylcypromine agreed to eat cheese for lunch, following which a continuous watch was kept on the blood pressure. For two hours the vigil was unrewarded, but within minutes of leaving the ward I was called back by a request to prescribe "aspirin for headache." On arrival, the patient was in the throes of a typical hypertensive crisis.

Coincidence continued to play a part. While walking down a Maudsley corridor one night, I was overtaken by the duty resident en route to a ward where two patients were simultaneously complaining of headache. Both had recently returned from the hospital cafeteria where cheese had just made its weekly appearance on the menu.

It was at this point that certainty dawned and created a restless inner tension, which is described as the "Eureka syndrome."[48] At this moment in the study it is possible to discern another feature common to the process of all discovery. It shows how a slender chain of coincidence can summate and interact with prior knowledge illustrating Louis Pasteur's aphorism that "Chance favors the prepared mind."[57] In this case, the preparedness was slight and the coincidences were substantial. The same mixture is always present, but the proportions differ according to whether the discovery arises from systematic study, chance, or serendipity.

SERENDIPITY

It would be pleasing to invoke serendipity[14,17,39,58-63] in this discovery, but to do so would overextend the idiom, even though serendipity is a word that will be much used during this meeting. Its most charming but erroneous definition is contained in the Zebulun column of the Archives of Internal Medicine, where it is stated to be "a portmanteau word signifying a mental state in which serenity and stupidity are blended . . . for example, the serendipity of a cow chewing its cud under a shady tree." [64]

The true origin has been traced by Theodore Remer in his book called *Serendipity*.[59] The word was coined by Horace Walpole in a letter to a friend written in 1754 and came from a Persian fairy tale called the "Three Princes of Serendip" (or Ceylon) whose heroes made fortunate discoveries by accident. The example selected by Walpole is that where one prince deduces that a mule, blind in the right eye, had travelled the same road frequently because the grass was eaten only on the left side of the path. Many important discoveries and most, if not all, those in biological psychiatry, came about in this way, probably the most striking being the monoamine oxidase inhibitors and LSD. The cheese story has nothing similar to relate except perhaps that writing a letter describing the syndrome produced a totally unexpected solution to the problem. This is reminiscent of Zebulun's other example of serendipity as being "the sort of thing that happens to you when on a dull day collecting fossils you find instead a beautiful woman who proves to be neither geologist nor archeologist." [64]

THE CLIMATE OF DISCOVERY

To cut short this digression, cases of hypertensive crisis now proved surprisingly easy to discover, and within six months 12 instances had been gathered, of whom eight had definitely eaten cheese within a short period of experiencing symptoms. These cases formed the basis of an article in the *Lancet*,[65] which still did not suffice to stifle skepticism. Many shared the opinion of one critic who found the whole concept "unscientific and premature," [66] a viewpoint supported by the observation that "everyone eats cheese" and that even those who had experienced one attack could eat it again with impunity. This unwillingness to accept a novel and apparently absurd observation is not new. In a small way, the idea that a common dietary substance might kill someone was as ridiculous as it once was to consider the earth round or that man was descended from a monkey. New ideas must fit what has been called "current common sense" [15] or the "cultural mentality" [39] of the time. This concept, which Goethe called the Zeitgeist,[15] includes all the conventions, technical abilities, and assumptions in which a scientific discovery must fit [14,17,32,67] unless a new conceptual framework is formulated to displace the old. This is a theme with broader implications for psychopharmacology. The many changes that occurred in biological psychiatry around 1954 [68] can be considered in such a light: the developments in biochemistry and neurophysiology before then had created both the plausible rationale to explain drug action as well as the more important climate of acceptance for the concept that mental illness might be biochemically determined and consequently reversed with drugs. At the same time, dissatisfaction with the older medications and the developing concepts of community care created a need for improvement that the new drugs fulfilled. This constellation of plausible rationale, acceptable climate, and widely felt need provided the Zeitgeist for chlorpromazine and much of what was to follow.

Most epochs of innovation are succeeded by the kind of slack interval in which we are currently becalmed. Today the Zeitgeist is somewhat different. It includes the current interest in so-called "nondrug factors," itself partly an expression of contemporary disillusion that could become a restraint on discovery unless we heed Hamilton's reminder [69] that such considerations apply only to small drugs and small illnesses. Another part of the contemporary Zeitgeist, with an alleged influence on the process of discovery, is the legislative strictures that are thought by some to restrain discovery by reducing the amount of new drug testing that is the seed bed of serendipity. It also follows that observations made at inclement times are either overlooked, ignored, or rejected.[17] Examples include Tyndall's discovery in 1857 of the antibacterial properties of penicillin, Mendel's genetic theories, and Semmelweis' discovery of puerperal fever.[3]

In the case of cheese, the Zeitgeist was altered by the observations of Professor Milne's unit [70] that a breakfast of Gorgonzola cheese was followed by appearance of tyramine in the body fluids, thus providing the necessary evidence, which in science precedes acceptance of an absurd idea. An increasing number of case reports began to appear together with one about a patient who had known of the association for several months, "but doctors laughed at the idea." [71]

That other clinicians quickly added reports will come as no surprise to those familiar with another general property of the discovery process: simultaneous observation. This is also an old topic of sociological inquiry. In 1922, William F. Ogburn and Dorothy S. Thomas compiled a list of 150 cases of multiple discoveries made independently by different scientists.[45] Dr. Elinor Barber and Dr. Robert Merton have since brought the subject up to date with an account of another 264 selected instances.[45] The appearance of all the new categories of drugs used in psychiatry between 1952 and 1960 is impressive testimony that the climate was ripe for innovation.

THE DISCOVERERS

That the socioscientific climate can play the major role in discovery is illustrated by Macaulay's often repeated aphorism that "without Columbus, America would have been discovered."[45] Certainly cheese was on the threshold of discovery when I stumbled across it in an academic milieu that combined the leisure to pursue a topic with the pressure to publish on it. Coincidence, with some personal credulity, curiosity, and impetuosity were the only individual ingredients. Discovery must often rest on such slender associations; this is not to deny the personal quality of those gifted individuals who make more important or repeated original observations. The characteristics of such creative scientists have been closely scrutinized by psychologists and sociologists. Guildford's factor analytic model of intelligence has isolated facets of problem-solving and creative ability distinct from other aspects of intelligence.[72] Among the three most commonly stressed aspects of creative thought have been an ability to see analogies[14,27,28] (or Koestler's bisociational thinking),[24] the tendency to seek original solutions[73] (the reverse of Karl Dunkar's "functional fixation") and a facility for a type of Gestalt thinking that sees parts in relation to the whole.[10,21] The way in which such capabilities fit within the actual process of discovery has also been clearly recorded[14,19,25,31,39] with the progression through a variable period of preparation, followed by a turmoil of seemingly unrelated fact, the inconsistency of which is often resolved in a final flash of insight (Geistesblitz)[3] that can occur at unexpected moments or even during sleep.[25,39] The example most often cited is Kekulé's dream,[14] where the cyclic nature of benzene presented itself during a dream in which wriggling snakes formed a ring by linking themselves head to tail. The mathmatician, Poincaré, who made many original discoveries, noted that such inspirations invariably follow on days of unfruitful work and later periods of apparent rest.[3]

The personality profile of 140 eminent research workers in physics, biology, and psychology were analyzed by Catell.[34] They differed significantly from normals at the 1% level by being more schizothymic, intelligent, dominant, but at the same time inhibited, emotionally sensitive, and radical in viewpoint. The biographical background of scientists has also been studied systematically by Taylor and Ellison[42] in an attempt to identify creative ability within the NASA organization by correlating predictions with performance. Wider ranging observations on creativity among scientists have been made by Anne Roe,[40] Margaret Mead,[74] and by Chambers,[35] who compared the life styles of 740 scientists divided into creative and uncreative groups. Initiative, dominance, and motivation represent the recurring theme with a lack of rigid religious affiliations. Unfortunately, it is this type of dominant personality and driving life style that also results in what Merton calls the "Matthew effect,"[47] after that verse in the Gospel: "For unto everyone that hath shall be given, and he shall have abundance." Such individuals attract young associates from whom they may usurp credit and coauthor unseen publications. In a psychosocial analysis, Merton identifies the characteristics of eminent men of science to whom this effect applies because their self-assurance leads them to search out risky but important problems and to highlight the results of their own inquiry.

ENCOURAGEMENT AND DISCOURAGEMENT IN DISCOVERY

Whatever the resources of the discoverer and however clement the times, every individual needs encouragement and must possess the fortitude to overcome discouragement. Even though the "cheese syndrome" was now firmly established, there remained a great deal that was unexplained, including the exact identification of the responsible amines and the reasons for variations in, or absence of, responses in different individuals. The dangerous nature of the reaction made animal research inevitable, and Sir Aubrey Lewis offered me the opportunity to work under Dr. Ted Marley in the pharmacology department at the Institute of Psychiatry. This opportunity was almost lost when the Professor of Pharmacology at Cambridge University declined to consider the topic suitable for a thesis on the grounds that the work would be best undertaken by a fully equipped pharmaceutical company.

It is common for novices to make discoveries, but this pattern of administrative response to an upstart's plea is another feature in the discovery process. More illustrious examples are provided by Sir Laurence Bragg's insistence that Crick and Watson discontinue their amateurish attempts to outdistance Linus Pauling [9] and by Professor Macleod's repeated refusal to allow Banting laboratory space to work on dogs until Macleod went on vacation to Scotland.[8] The fact that on his return Macleod assumed much of the credit and later accepted a share in the Nobel Prize for discovering insulin is a cogent example of the Matthew effect in action. This resistance to new ideas ("functional fixation") may be one aspect of the difference between age and youth that helps to account for the fact that over 80% of the world's leading discoveries were made by men between the ages of 25 and 45.[5] William Harvey anticipated the generation gap when he remarked that no one over 40 ever accepted or understood the circulation of the blood,[14] and Sir William Osler referred to one of his harmless obsessions as a conviction concerning the "comparative uselessness of men above forty years of age." [75] He deduced this opinion (as others have done) [14] from the observation that discoveries in medicine almost always came from men "on whose back the sun was still shining" in what he called the "anabolic and constructive" period between 25 and 40.

PRIORITY AND CRYPTOMNESIA IN DISCOVERY

In our particular instance, resistance was easily overcome when Dr. Marley interceded successfully with the University, and work on animals was then ready to begin. I had survived apprenticeship as an intern to a future President of the Royal College of Surgeons without ever learning to tie a surgical knot, but under Dr. Marley's patient tutelage and with the daily sacrifice of five or six animals, I eventually learned to set up a pithed rat, to cannulate its carotid artery, and even to develop a means of injecting homogenized cheese into the duodenum. As these techniques were about mastered, we learned that the pharmaceutical company with whom we had discussed our first results had reneged on an understanding to publish simultaneously by submitting a preliminary communication to the *Lancet*. For several weeks we worked late, surrounded by cages of cats, rats, pigeons, and hens in the crowded inadequate conditions that English research workers take perverse pride in. Eventually, the two preliminary publications appeared together.[76,77] The race for priority is an unwelcome side effect of the Zeitgeist and its resulting phenomenon of multiple discovery which, contrary to popular opinion, is declining in frequency and acerbity. Since original observation is the raison d'etre of science, it follows that conflict over priority has always been an "integral part of the relations between scientists." [44] Merton has chronicled many irate exchanges between the giants of old, beginning with Galileo, who inveighs against an unspecified villain who "attempted to rob me of that glory which was mine" [44] and extending on through Newton, Faraday, Darwin, and many others. Failure to achieve priority or recognition has also been shown to produce devastating effects on the productivity of individual scientists. Semmelweis, who anticipated Lister and Pasteur, was spurned by his colleagues and ended his days insane.[14]

The ambivalence created by the dilemma of claiming priority and remaining modest is considerable both for scientists themselves and their biographers. Merton [46] provides two examples that are especially pertinent to the topic and setting of this conference. He comments on Ernest Jones' erroneous statement that Freud was "never interested in questions of priority" by dissecting out 150 examples from Freud's work including a dream that Freud himself interprets as an expression of regret that he lost priority in the discovery of cocaine to his colleague Koller by postponing some experiments in order to visit his fiancée. Cocaine was the subject of a similar discrepancy between the facts and the biographer of that great Baltimore surgeon, William Halsted. The same book that maintains he was "indifferent to matters of priority" contains a letter from Halsted to a friend complaining that "I showed Wölfler how to use cocaine. He had declared it was useless in surgery, but before I left Vienna, he published an enthusiastic article in one of the daily papers on the subject. It did not, however, occur to him to mention my name." The practice of establishing priority through the newspapers is not entirely unheard of even today.

The only satisfactory solution to the personal conflict and interpersonal friction created by this ambivalent situation is the type of honest admission made by Charles Darwin [44] that "My love of natural science had been much aided by the ambition to be esteemed by my fellow naturalists." In a similar vein, Hans Selye [78] was still more explicit when he noted, "All the scientists I know sufficiently well to judge (and I include myself in this group) are extremely anxious to have their work recognized and approved by others. Is it not below the dignity of an objective scientific mind to permit such a distortion of his true motives? Besides, what is there to be ashamed of?"

With hindsight, I wonder whether the pharmacist, G. E. F. Rowe, who really discovered the cheese reaction, has received the recognition he deserves. Although he is mentioned in several of our articles and was sent all of them at the conclusion of our four years' work, he was not named in the first paper, which established priority, and only one textbook of psychopharmacology makes correct attribution.[79]

In the same tenor, there is another adverse effect of the discovery process called "cryptomnesia."[44] The term designates unconscious plagiary and is related to selective forgetting. There are many examples in the literature including the publication by two eminent poets of the same poem, one of whom had read the other's work years previously and then suppressed the fact.[15] Darwin made a point of recording unfavorable data because he forgot them more readily.[14] Three years after the original patient who ate cheese was described, I met again the hospital detail man who visited the Maudsley at that time. Our reminiscence revealed how much of his own contribution and encouragement had been usurped or forgotten and how much justifiable resentment he felt over a complete failure to acknowledge that debt even in a footnote. It was later repaid by a joint publication[80] describing some of the earlier steps in the discovery, and I now have his gift at home of a cheese board engraved with the well-remembered and discouraging phrase, "everyone eats cheese."

MULTIDISCIPLINARY DIVERSIONS IN DISCOVERY

Soon after the animal research was running smoothly, another dietary precipitant was rediscovered. The first 12 cases[65] included one patient who had eaten a proprietary yeast extract called "Marmite," which is a sticky brown residue aptly described by an American colleague as a sort of "slum gullion." It is used as a sandwich spread or dissolved in water as a beverage and is popular in hospitals on account of a high vitamin B content. Nothing had been done to investigate this substance in animals until we were telephoned by a London general practitioner. His patient had experienced several hypertensive episodes due to cheese and had been advised by her psychiatrist to replace this favorite article of diet with "Marmite." On doing so she again experienced the typical symptoms of severe headache.[81] It was a simple matter to inject "Marmite" into a rat and observe the large increase in blood pressure after a monoamine oxidase inhibitor. This same patient subsequently volunteered for a series of carefully controlled experiments on the Maudsley Hospital metabolic ward, in which it was possible to show the subtle influence of dosage and timing of medication on severity of the hypertension caused by "Marmite."[2] There is one other digression relevant to the process of discovery. The general practitioner who rediscovered "Marmite" was Dr. Anthony Ryle, who has carried out much original research into psychosocial problems in general practice. His father was Dr. John Ryle, Professor of Social Medicine at the University of Oxford. In preparing this lecture, I read again the chapter on Research in Clinical Medicine that is part of the elder Ryle's well-known textbook the *Natural History of Disease*.[82] In that chapter, Ryle discusses choice of candidates for research scholarships and mentions that "a scholarly heredity should, by Galtonian doctrine, be considered a very distinct advantage." Perhaps this was why, out of the many thousands of general practitioners around London, it was his son who noticed "Marmite," who knew someone else was interested, and took the trouble to communicate his observation. The lineage of distinguished scientists like the Huxleys certainly supports the older Ryle's contention of genetic continuity in research ability.[33]

Our research now extended not only to other species, but into other disciplines.[83-88] This included collaboration with Dr. Mabbitt, a microbiologist at the National Institute of Research in Dairying, to determine the amine composition of different cheeses and the factors that influenced their production.[83] Chromatographic work there also showed that there were large amounts of histamine in "Marmite," which led in turn to advice on modification in its manufacturing process.[84] There was much interesting basic pharmacology accomplished on the interaction between these amines and the monoamine oxidase inhibitors and their joint effects on the cardiovascular alpha and beta receptors.[87] In addition, there were more light-hearted digressions. We exploded the myth that only cheeses with visible and olfactory evidence of putrefaction contained amines, and discovered that apparently similar pieces of cheese may differ constitutionally like one pile of garbage from the next.[88]

SUPPORT FOR DISCOVERY

All this demonstrates both the large number of avenues that open up from a new area of research and the interdisciplinary nature of the effort that is nowadays required to exploit them. In one area of physical research, the number of papers with a solitary author dropped from 93% before 1920 to only 28% after 1940.[46] Those whose purpose is to support and encourage the process of discovery know what problems this interdisciplinary factor poses in the design of teaching and research organizations and in their funding and support. There has been much discussion of the role of government [17, 89, 90] and the merits of institutions with single-minded aims versus departments with what Bean described as "a propinquity of persons with a bewildering diversity of interests." [91] My own experience was possibly fortunate but seems to illustrate that a mission-oriented individual can usually find the encouragement and help needed from both sources. From a government paid clinical post, I was able to enter the broadly based research Institute of Psychiatry and to collaborate with the more specialized National Institute of Research in Dairying. For a time, support also came in a Fellowship from the independent and publically funded Mental Health Research Fund.

ADUMBRATION OF DISCOVERY

When the pieces of the whole process of this discovery were finally assembled, after nearly four years of work in man and animals, they provided an explanation to many of the earlier illogicalities.[2] They also invoke one final comment on the general process of discovery, which has been called "adumbrationism." [45] This is the minimization of a finding by the suggestion that it has been anticipated. While this is clearly a vice when discussing the work of others, it may be permissible and even salutary in considering one's own, particularly if the discovery relates to a potentially lethal and entirely preventable side effect. Hippocrates himself expressed some doubts about cheese [92]: "It is not enough to know that cheese is a bad article of food in that it gives pain to anyone eating it in excess, but what sort of pain, and why, and with what principle in man it disagrees. . . ." In the process of our search we rediscovered that tyrosine was named after the Greek word for cheese from which the amino acid was first isolated in 1846 [93]; that tyramine was discovered to be a hypertensive agent by Sir Henry Dale and his colleague, Dixon, in 1909 [94]; and that two years later Findlay,[95] who used it in early experiments with the sphygmomanometer, predicted that the rises in blood pressure it produced might cause cerebral hemorrhage. We found also that monoamine oxidase had been originally named tyramine oxidase after its first known substrate [96] and that the role of this enzyme in the gut and liver was thought by Blaschko [97] in 1952 to include the denial of access to the circulation of amines in foodstuffs. Worse still, severe throbbing headache and hypertension were noted to occur in four out of 42 tuberculosis patients by Ogilvie [98] in 1955 during one of the first trials of iproniazid in England. Another 40 cases, including several deaths, occurred between then and the incrimination of cheese in 1963.

CONCLUSION

Finally, I would like to return to the main purpose of this symposium. The importance of a need to understand and encourage the discovery process is often expressed. A 1957 issue of the *Journal of the American Medical Association* contained two articles on the topic,[61, 63] one of which selected iproniazid as an example of a drug that was "baffling researchers with its versatility." [61] An accompanying editorial [62] questioned whether "little boy curiosity," might either be cultivated into a permanent asset or dulled by a welter of "not to be questioned fact." The possibility of detecting and encouraging scientific creativity has been widely studied.[10, 30, 41, 43, 73, 99-105] Those who are skeptical of such ambitious aims might share the view of an eminent English inventor [106] that discovery is not taught but only nurtured by apprenticeship and who supported this view with the comforting thought that "if you're there first, you have nothing to read. You've got all your time to think." A cautionary note was also sounded by Lawrence Kubie [107] in an analysis of unsolved problems in the scientific career. He questions whether students should best be warned that scientific success is often determined by social forces outside individual creative capacity and will to work hard. The frustrated urge to discover might breed a generation of cynical, amoral, and disillusioned young scientists who suffer from what he calls a "new psychosocial ailment which may not be wholly unrelated to the gangster tradition of dead-end kids."

Perhaps such a warning is timely for younger psychopharmacologists. There have been no outstanding new discoveries for 10 years, and the excitement of two decades past has given way to a more critical and iconoclastic spirit. In drawing attention to Kubie's fears, Merton [44] has provided a solution by pointing out that for "most of us artisans of research, getting things into print becomes a symbolic equivalent for making a new discovery."

The educational hopes for this symposium are coupled with its intention to commend those who have made pioneer discoveries in biological psychiatry. It casts a modest perspective on that purpose to recall Sir Aubrey Lewis's admonition [108]:

> We are not living through a period that marks a new epoch; there is no Galileo or Darwin, no Harvey or Newton in psychiatry and psychology, nor to put our aspirations on a more realistic plane, have there been discoveries during the last 20 years comparable to those that have signalled the growth of therapeutics and surgery in other fields. Psychiatric advances have been less dramatic and less conclusive. Still, to those who have taken part in them, they have given the satisfaction and excited the hopes out of which enthusiasm is generated.

I am sure that our enthusiasm and hopes for the future of biological psychiatry will be excited by the accounts of past discovery that are about to unfold.

Acknowledgment. Like the discovery it reports, this paper leans heavily on the work, encouragement, and support of others. In particular, I thank Dr. William Bean and Dr. Robert Merton for providing source material and Dr. Irving A. Taylor for an extensive bibliography on creativity. Miss Gertrude Bloomer kindly assisted in the collection of material.

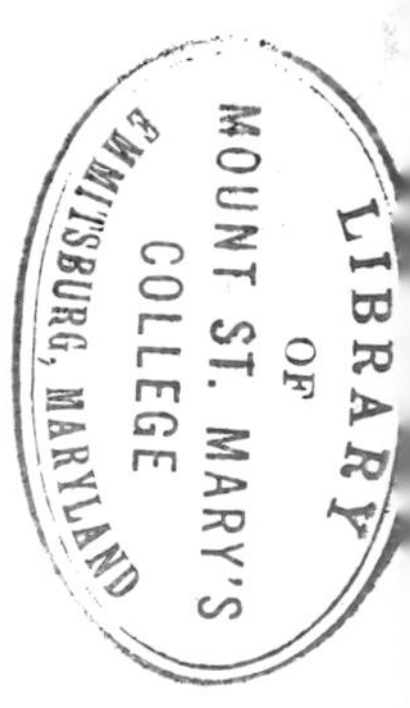

REFERENCES

1. Mayo, W.: Remarks on the romance of medicine, Mayo Clin Proc *10*:393-394, 1935.

2. Blackwell, B., Marley, E., Price, J., and Taylor, D.: Hypertensive interactions between monoamine oxidase inhibitors and foodstuffs, Brit J Psychiat *113*:349-365, 1967.

3. Taton, R.: Reason and Chance in Scientific Discovery, New York, Philosophical Library, 1957.

4. Lipetz, Ben-Ami: A Guide to Case Studies of Scientific Activity, Carlisle (Mass), Intermedia, Inc., 1965.

5. Garrett, A. B.: The Flash of Genius, Princeton (NJ), Van Nostrand, 1963.

6. Andrade, E. N., daC.: Sir Isaac Newton: His Life and Work, New York, Doubleday and Anchor Books, 1958.

7. Carter, R.: Breakthrough: The Saga of Jonas Salk, New York, Trident, 1966.

8. Harris, S.: Banting's Miracle, Philadelphia, Lippincott, 1946.

9. Watson, J. D.: The Double Helix, New York, Atheneum, 1968.

10. Wertheimer, M.: Productive Thinking, New York, Harper, 1959.

11. Dubos, R. J.: Louis Pasteur: Freelance of Science, Boston, Little, 1950.

12. Marquardt, M.: Paul Ehrlich, London, Heinemann, 1949.

13. Alamshah, W. W.: The conditions for creativity, J Creative Behav *1*:305, 1967.

14. Beveridge, W. I. B.: The Art of Scientific Investigation, New York, Norton, 1957.

15. Boring, E. G.: Psychological factors in the scientific process, Amer Sci *42*:639-645, 1954.

16. Cannon, W. B.: The Way of an Investigator, New York, Norton, 1945.

17. Cohen, I. B.: Science, Servant of Man, Boston, Little, 1948.

18. Davies, J. T.: The Scientific Approach, London, Acad Press, 1965.

19. Ghiselin, B., ed.: The Creative Process, New York, Mentor, 1955.

20. Golann, S. E.: Psychological study of creativity, Psychol Bull *60*:548-565, 1963.

21. Hanson, N. R.: Patterns of Discovery, New York, Cambridge, 1958.

22. Hinton, B. L.: Environmental frustration and creative problem solving, J Appl Psychol *52*:211-217, 1968.

23. Ingle, D. J.: Principles of Research in Biology and Medicine, Philadelphia, Lippincott, 1958.

24. Koestler, A.: The Act of Creation, New York, Macmillan, 1964.

25. Lewin, B. D.: Remarks on creativity, imagery and the dream, J Nerv Ment Dis *149*:115-121, 1960.

26. McGhee, Paul A., and Coler, Myron, A., eds.: Essays on Creativity in the Sciences, New York, NYU, 1963.

27. Mednick, S. A.: The associative basis of the creative process, Psychol Rev *69*:220-232, 1962.

28. Shapiro, R. J.: The integrating of remotely associated concepts as a process in scientific creativity, Psychol Afr *11*:40-48, 1965.

29. Tatum, E. L.: A case history in biological research, Science *129*:1711-1715, 1959.

30. Taylor, D. W.: Thinking and creativity, Ann NY Acad Sci *91*:108-127, 1960.

31. Wallas, G.: The Art of Thought, New York, Harcourt, 1926.

32. Wightman, W. P. D.: The Growth of Scientific Ideas, New Haven (Conn), Yale, 1951.

33. Brain, R.: Some Reflections on Genius, Philadelphia, Lippincott, 1960.

34. Cattell, R. B.: The personality and motivation of the researcher from measurements of contemporaries and from biography, *in* Taylor, Calvin W., and Barron, Frank, eds.: Scientific Creativity: Its Recognitions and Development, New York, Wiley, 1963.

35. Chambers, J. A.: Creative scientists of today, Science *145*:1203-1205, 1964.

36. Foster, F. P.: The human relations of creative individuals, J Creative Behav *2*:111, 1968.

37. Fox, H. H.: A critique on creativity in scientists, *in* Coler, Myron A., and McGhee, Paul A., eds.: Essays on Creativity in the Sciences, New York, NYU, 1963.

38. Guilford, J. P.: Intellectual resources and their values as seen by scientists, *op. cit.*, ref. 34.

39. Porterfield, A. L.: Creative Factors in Scientific Research, Durham (NC), Duke, 1941.

40. Roe, A.: The Making of a Scientist, New York, Dodd, 1952.

41. Taylor, C. W., and Barron, F., eds.: Scientific Creativity: Its Recognition and Development, New York, Wiley, 1963.

42. Taylor, C. W., and Ellison, R. L.: Biographical predicators of scientific performance, Science *155:*1075-1080, 1967.

43. Thurstone, L. L.: The scientific study of inventive talent, *in* Parnes, S. J., and Harding, H. F., eds.: A Source Book for Creative Thinking, New York, Scribner's, 1962.

44. Merton, R. K.: Priorities in scientific discovery: A chapter in the sociology of science, Amer Sociol Rev *22:*635-659, 1957.

45. ——: Singletons and multiples in scientific discovery: A chapter in the sociology of science, Proc Amer Philosophical Soc *105:*472-486, 1961.

46. ——: Resistance to the systematic study of multiple discoveries in science, Europ J Sociol *4:*237-282, 1963.

47. ——: The Matthew effect in science, Science *159:*56-63, 1968.

48. ——: Behavior patterns of scientists, Amer Sci *57:*1-23, 1969.

49. Aldridge, M., and Oakley, N.: Tranylcypromine, Lancet *2:*932, 1961.

50. Bass, B. H.: *Ibid.*, p. 1099.

51. Dally, P. J.: Fatal reactions associated with tranylcypromine and methamphetamine, Lancet *1:*123, 1962.

52. Dormer, A. E.: Side effects of tranylcypromine, Lancet *T:*162, 1962.

53. McLure, J. L.: Reactions associated with tranylcypromine, Lancet *1:*1351, 1962.

54. Mason, A.: Fatal reactions associated with tranylcypromine and methamphetamine, *Ibid.*, p. 1073.

55. Rae, J. W., and Harriman, B. P.: Tranylcypromine, *Ibid.*, p. 162.

56. Blackwell, B.: Tranylcypromine, Lancet *1:*168, 1963

57. Vallery-Radot, R.: The Life of Pasteur, Trans. R. L. Devonshire, New York, Doubleday, 1924.

58. Bean, W. B.: Serendipity, Curr Med Digest (May):679-680, 1967.

59. Remer, T. G.: Serendipity and the Three Princes, Norman (Okla), Univ Okla, 1965.

60. Zebulun Column: Serendipity, Arch Intern Med (Chicago) *112:*785-787, 1963.

61. Golin, M.: Serendipity—big word in medical progress, JAMA *165:* 2084-2087, 1957.

62. Editorial: "Medicine's 'Happy Accidents'," *Ibid.*, pp. 2088-2089.

63. Compere, E. L.: Research, serendipity, and orthopedic surgery, *Ibid.*, pp. 2070-2073.

64. Zebulun Column: Serendipity, Arch Intern Med (Chicago) *111:*385-386, 1963.

65. Blackwell, B.: Hypertensive crisis due to monoamine oxidase inhibitors, Lancet *2:*849-851, 1963.

66. Weber, J. C. P.: Tranylcypromine and cheese, *Ibid.*, p. 587.

67. Richards, D. W.: A clinician's view of advances in therapeutics, *in* Talalay, Paul, ed.: Drugs in Our Society, Baltimore, Johns Hopkins, 1963.

68. Lape, E. E., ed.: Evolving role of government in research in the United States and unsolved clinical problems: Schizophrenia, *in* Medical Research: A

Mid-Century Survey (The American Foundation), Cambridge (Mass), Riverside, 1955.

69. Hamilton, M.: *In* Rickels, Karl, ed.: Non-Specific Factors in Drug Therapy, Springfield (Ill), Thomas, 1968, pp. 133-135.

70. Asatoor, A. M., Levi, A. J., and Milne, M. D.: Tranylcypromine and cheese, Lancet *2:*733-734, 1963.

71. Read, A. E. A., and Arora, B.: Tranylcypromine, *Ibid.*, p. 587.

72. Guilford, J. P.: Intelligence has three facets, Science *160:*615-620, 1968.

73. Maltzman, I., Simon, S., Raskin, D., and Licht, L.: Experimental studies in the training of originality, Psychol Monogr *74:*(6), 1960.

74. Mead, M.: *In* Anderson, H. H., ed.: Creativity and Its Cultivation, New York, Harper, 1959.

75. Osler, Sir William: Aequanimitas, Philadelphia, Blakiston, 1932.

76. Blackwell, B., and Marley, E.: Interaction between cheese and monoamine oxidase inhibitors in rats and cats, Lancet *1:*530-531, 1964.

77. Natoff, I. L.: Cheese and monoamine oxidase inhibitors: (Interactions in anesthetized cats), *Ibid.*, pp. 532-533.

78. Selye, H.: The Stress of Life, New York, McGraw-Hill, 1956.

79. Klein, D. F., and Davis, J. M.: Diagnosis and Drug Treatment of Psychiatric Disorders, Baltimore, Williams & Wilkins, 1969.

80. Samuel, G., and Blackwell, B.: Monoamine oxidase inhibitors and cheese: A process of discovery, Hosp Med 2(#8):942-943, 1968.

81. Blackwell, B., Marley, E., and Ryle, A.: Hypertensive crisis associated with monoamine oxidase inhibitors, Lancet *T:*722-723, 1964.

82. Ryle, J. A.: The Natural History of Disease, New York, Oxford, 1948, p. 445.

83. Blackwell, B., and Mabbitt, L. A.: Tyramine in cheese related to hypertensive crises after monoamine oxidase inhibitors, Lancet *1:*938-940, 1965.

84. Blackwell, B., Mabbitt, L. A., and Marley, E.: Histamine and tyramine content of yeast products, J Food Sci *34:*47-51, 1969.

85. Blackwell, B., and Marley, E.: Interactions of cheese and its constituents with monoamine oxidase inhibitors, Brit J Pharmacol *26:*120-141, 1966a.

86. ——: Interactions of yeast extracts and their constituents with monoamine oxidase inhibitors, Brit J Pharmacol *26:*142-161, 1966b.

87. ——: Depressor effects with sympathomimetic amines after blockade of cardiovascular α-receptors, Nature *213:*840, 1967.

88. ——: Monoamine oxidase inhibitors and intolerance to foodstuffs, Bibl Nutr Dieta *11:*96-110, 1968.

89. Himsworth, Sir Harold: Administration and the structure of scientific knowledge, Brit Med J *4:*517-522, 1969.

90. Stewart, W. H.: Research and public responsibility, *in* Lyght, Charles E., ed.: Reflections on Research and the Future of Medicine, New York, McGraw-Hill, 1967.

91. Bean, W. B.: Institutes versus departments, Curr Med Digest (Mar): 277-279, 1968.

92. Brock, A. J.: Greek Medicine, London, Dent & Sons, 1929, p. 49.

93. Liebig, J.: Baldriansaure Und Ein Neuer Korper aus Kasetoff, Ann d Chem *57:*127-129, 1846.

94. Dale, H. H., and Dixon, W. E.: Action of pressor amines produced by putrefaction, J Physiol (London) *39:*25-44, 1909.

95. Findlay, L.: The systolic pressure at different points of the circulation in the child and the adult, Quart J Med *4:*489-497, 1911.

96. Hare, M. L. C.: Tyramine oxidase; new enzyme system in liver, Biochem J *22:*968-979, 1928.

97. Blaschko, H.: Amine oxidase and amine metabolism, Pharmacol Rev *4*:415-458, 1952.

98. Ogilvie, C.: The treatment of pulmonary tuberculosis with iproniazid and isoniazid, Quart J Med *24*:175-289, 1955.

99. Brown, A. E.: Creativity can be stimulated, Chem Eng News *38*(43): 102-110, 1960.

100. Getzels, J. W., and Jackson, P. W.: Creativity and Intelligence: Explorations with Gifted Children, New York, Wiley, 1962.

101. Mackinnon, D. W.: The nature and nurture of creative talent, Amer Psychol *17*:484-495, 1962.

102. Smith, R. F.: The deliberate induction of new ideas, *op. cit.*, ref. 37.

103. Steiner, G. A., ed.: The Creative Organization, Chicago, Univ of Chicago, 1965.

104. Taylor, D. W., Berry, R. C., and Block, C. H.: Does group participation when using brainstorming facilitate or inhibit creative thinking?, Administrative Sci Quart *3*:23, 1958.

105. Torrance, P. E.: Guiding Creative Talent, New Jersey, Prentice Hall, 1962.

106. Williams, F. C.: How to invent, Int Sci Technology (Feb):49-53, 1964.

107. Kubie, L. S.: Some unsolved problems of the scientific career, Amer Sci *42*:104-112, 1954.

108. Lewis, Sir Aubrey: Medicine and the affections of the mind, Brit Med J *2*:1549-1557, 1963.

CHAPTER

2

Psychopharmacology: On Beginning in a New Science

PERSONAL RECOLLECTIONS

JOEL ELKES, MD *

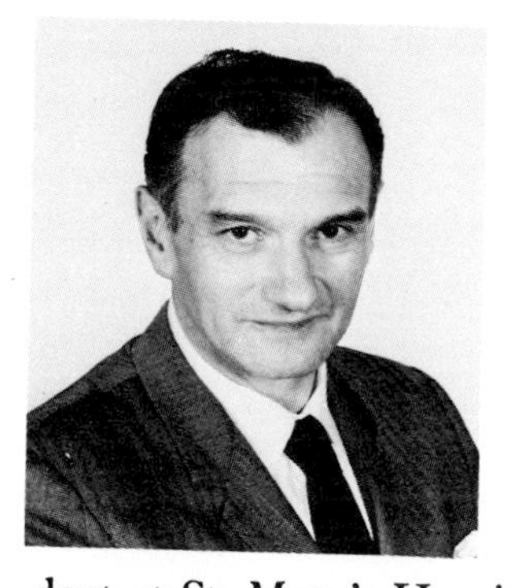

IT IS A RARE OCCASION that affords one the privilege to reminisce in company such as this. One cherishes such occasions. The Editor has encouraged me to be "personal": and here, more or less, is how things went with me.

AN ODD BEGINNING

On a particular afternoon in the summer of 1934, while a medical student at St. Mary's Hospital, London, I was having tea and anchovy toast with my erstwhile chief, Dr. Alastair Frazer. We talked about physiology in general, and his field in particular. Alastair was working on the absorption of fat from the alimentary canal, in which field he later became a world authority. He was especially concerned with the chylomicron, a physiologically present particle, flooding the circulation from the thoracic duct after a fatty meal. He asked me to peer down a microscope; and there, under dark ground illumination, I saw the mysterious dance of the particles in Brownian movement. This touched me deeply. What manner of bodies were they? I knew that I could get interested in studying the properties

* Director, Department of Psychiatry and Behavioral Sciences, The Johns Hopkins University School of Medicine, Psychiatrist-in-chief, the Johns Hopkins Hospital, Baltimore.

of these bodies, particularly the constitution of their envelope giving them their electric charge. Microelectrophoresis and various flocculation techniques came to mind. I suppose that what intrigued me then (and still intrigues me) was inferring the properties of a structure from physicochemical measurements, building up a mental picture on the basis of collateral evidence. This wish to visualize has stayed with me throughout my life. My imaginings, I find, are always very approximate and qualitative. I have to carry some kind of map (quite often a wrong map) of things in my head. Playing with macromolecular configurations became quite a hobby with me in those days. In any event, with the chylomicron, and with its lipoproteins, my quest into the interface between physical chemistry and biology began. I started to read physical chemistry voraciously. I suppose it was the sense of penetrating and getting to the fundamental building blocks of life that drove me. It was, of course, the pursuit of an illusion; but even then, the sense of pattern, of configuration, of subtle variations of an arrangement and charge distribution, haunted one. I loved reading Irving Langmuir's introductory lectures on the deposition of gaseous films on metals. I went to Sir Eric Rideal's laboratory in the Department of Colloid Science, Cambridge, and met Shulman, Alexander, Crisp and others who had taken Langmuir's work (and the "Langmuir trough") a long way as a technique for studying cohesion among the asymmetric molecules, including lipid/protein interaction. I loved this clean visualizable technique for measuring the forces and electric charges operating in monomolecular films; and was incidentally tremendously taken with Eric Rideal's ironic ways as a laboratory director. I developed a microelectrophoretic cell with which I used to study the mobility of chylomicrons in an electric field by direct observation under a dark ground microscope; and indeed had the curious satisfaction of finding that paper [1] quoted in Starling's *Principles of Human Physiology* before I finished medical school; though this was less due to the distinction of the paper than to the sheer length of time, which, for various reasons, I took to finish medical school.

Thus, my having once tasted of it, the mystery of lipoprotein structure took hold. In 1942, Alastair Frazer invited me to join him in starting a Department of Pharmacology in Birmingham, England. Birmingham, even then, had the makings of the great university which it has since become. For one thing, it had a splendid campus, all compact. Within five minutes' walk of the medical school and hospital were the basic science Departments of Chemistry and Physics. Conversation at lunch was propitious, and soon turned to lipoproteins. The structure of liquid crystals, the nature of forces, polar, nonpolar and steric, the bonding that made for their ordered cohesion, their ability to interact with water and ions continued to excite. I found myself visualizing these structures, streaming through their pores like a sodium ion, negotiating various channels and portals with chains collapsing spring-like as these tiny compartments opened and closed. I was influenced tremendously in this respect by Astbury, who was just coming into his own at Leeds, and who was anticipating "molecular biology" by a full two decades, by Albert Szent-Gyorgyi, and by Dervichian of the Pasteur Institute, whom I remember playing with molecular models on the floor, as a child does with toys. And then one day I suddenly realized that the nervous system was full of lipoproteins, and that myelin was a highly ordered lipoprotein structure.

I came upon the papers of Francis Schmitt [2,3] who was then at St. Louis. I wrote to him, and got back a handsome collection of reprints describing his work on the structure of the myelin sheath. I was fascinated by his structural diagrams. Here was a highly ordered, esthetically beautiful arrangement, which fitted the facts and which made it possible to consider the way in which bimolecular leaflets were built into a highly specialized organ, the cell membrane, which was ion sensitive, and specifically electrochemically responsive. Myelin, I thought, could provide a fine model for the understanding of the structure of membranes. I was convinced of that; so was my friend Alastair Frazer; but I found it hard to convince others. However, one fine thing happened: Bryan Finean walked into my laboratory as my first PhD student.

Bryan was a red-headed, taciturn, tough little Irishman, given to the singing of Gregorian chants on his days off, who had got his degree in chemistry doing crystallography of the traditional kind. He was so reluctant to push himself forward that I was not even sure, when we discussed working arrangements, whether we would get on, and do anything. But as we got talking about the crystallography of macromolecules in living systems, as we looked at Francis Schmitt's reprints, we began to get excited about the possibility of applying low-angle x-ray diffraction to these systems. There were great technical difficulties in those days—the low power of the local x-ray tubes, the length of exposure; also, camera slits and collimators were all unsuitable. But one afternoon Bryan brought back his first successful x-ray diffraction photograph of dry nerve, showing clearly the Schmitt dimensions. Things obviously were possible, even with local equipment; and we were off. To me there was also a profound, personal and psychological element in this engagement. I was moving away from somebody else's field, and entering a field that somehow mysteriously pulled me—the nervous system; albeit by way of creeping up the myelin sheath! What happened out of this collaboration is on record.[4-6]

For one thing, Finean and I clarified some of the factors governing protein-lipid interaction. For another, we began a series of x-ray diffraction studies on the living, irrigated frog nerve, which to the best of my knowledge were the first of their kind. These experiments, which examined the effects of moisture, temperature, alcohol and ether on myelin structure, brought Finean rapid recognition, credit being due him in fullest measure. For it was he who developed specialized cells, who devised special slits and collimators. When the local x-ray tube gave out, we moved to the crystallographic laboratory of the Royal Institution, London, using the tube that J. D. Bernal had used for his famous early work. Gradually, in a small circle of physical chemists, and what was then the nucleus of molecular biology in Britain, we made some headway. However, when we demonstrated our findings to the Physiological or the Pharmacological Society, we got very peculiar looks. Nobody knew what we were up to; and people were very skeptical of the model value of the myelin for the study of the structure of biological membranes. Today, of course, it is different; and I am pleased to find our diagrams copied in textbooks and journals[7,8]; but in those days, only a few stopped by our demonstration stalls in the Physiological Society. It is significant who they were: Lord Adrian, Sir Henry Dale, J. H. Gaddum and Alan Hodgkin. They were interested. So was Astbury, so was Bernal; and as Bryan Finean's work was recognized, as he went to MIT, to Caracas, to Stockholm, as he published his monographs (including one with Engstrom),[9,10] his views gathered strength. Today he is a widely recognized and internationally respected authority, and I am glad for him, and a little proud at having had something to do with his success.

For me there was also a much more personal satisfaction. I was in the nervous system, and vastly attracted by it. Yet, as it is apparent, one still edged safely at the periphery. Myelin to be sure was the nervous system; but it was quite a way from behavior and the mode of action of psychoactive drugs; in fact, one could hardly be further away. Yet it is this work with Finean that led me into the nervous system, but not before another lucky circumstance had cleared the way.

PHARMACOLOGY AND EXPERIMENTAL PSYCHIATRY IN BIRMINGHAM, ENGLAND

There was in Birmingham, in the laboratory immediately below the Department of Pharmacology, a small subdepartment administered by the Dean's office, called Mental Diseases Research. In charge of it was a gifted neuropathologist, Dr. Pickworth, who held the view that mental disease was a capillary disease, and that all disorders were reflected in an abnormal cerebral vascular bed. He had developed beautiful benzidine staining techniques for demonstrating the small cerebral vessels; and the laboratory was filled with innumerable slices and slides of the brain in all manner of pathological states, stained by his methods. This treasury represented Dr. Pickworth's life work. However, he retired soon after I came on the scene; and his place was taken by a gifted, elegant Viennese colleague, Dr. Franz Schütz. When I look back, I conclude that Franz Schütz, possibly unaware of it himself, became an agent in my very fate. For he was working on some aspects of brain physiology and drug action. He was highly original in his methods, and developed foam adsorption techniques for the fractionation of cerebral metabolites. He was enormously industrious, and given to hours and hours of voluble talk. As I listened to him, and as I read on the topics he was working in (e.g., the *in vivo* formation of aldehydes and the metabolism of barbiturates), I got a sense of exhilaration and excitement. For here, actually, in a laboratory a floor below my own, was somebody working on the chemistry of the brain, on the intermediate metabolism of drugs affecting mental function. Mental disease research was not an exercise in futility, but actually possible, actually taking place; I pressed for more direct access.

Here serendipity took a part again; for as Dr. Pickworth resigned, the laboratory reverted to the Department of Pharmacology, and I became administratively responsible for its conduct. Our Department of Pharmacology was growing by leaps and bounds. When we arrived in Birmingham, there were two people; when I left, in 1950, there were 42 in the department. I was getting my taste for administration, and helping people to perform. While I was busying myself with Bryan Finean, and talking to Franz Schütz, another event took place. The war had ended. Our Military Intelligence had given us insights into the secret German chemical warfare work, and particularly the anticholinesterases and their tremendous specificity for certain enzymes in the brain. We were asked to work with the anticholinesterases: DFP, TEPP, and the like. We started mapping the cholinesterases in various areas of the brain; inhibiting the "true" and "pseudo" enzymes from birth; observing the effect of such inhibition on the emergence of various inborn reflexes.[11, 12] It was a long, long way from fat absorption, and some way from lipoproteins. But, at long last, it was brain; it was drugs; and I was even beginning to "smell" that mysterious entity called behavior. In those days, there were no texts on neurochemistry. There was Page's book [13]; there were Quastel's papers [14]; there were Harold Himwich's and Derek Richter's great early contributions [15,16]; and there was, of course, always Thudichum.[17] These I could read. I started also reading Masserman [18] and McDougall.[19] And then there appeared, in 1948, Feldberg and Vogt's classic paper in the *Journal of Physiology* [20] questioning the universal role of acetylcholine.

In retrospect, it becomes apparent to me that I was once again approaching my central interest, gingerly and carefully, as if I were defusing a bomb; for it is plain to me that what attracted me to mental disease research was an urge to leave the bench and get to people; and what made me circumambulate this purpose was my feeling of safety with things. Somehow, mental disease research, or experimental psychiatry (as I was beginning to call it in my mind), presented a sort of compromise. It led inevitably to human work, but it did so by way of experiment and control. This self-deception worked for a time, for an astonishingly long time; it took a further five years to break through it.

We were, then, beginning to feel our way with the anticholinesterases; and at the opposite pole I began to read widely on the psychoactive drugs. The first required dissection and mapping of the distribution of enzymes in various parts of the brain—a regional neurochemical approach; the other, the human experiment. Kluver's papers on mescaline [21] proved an illumination. Here was perception, clarity, depth, humanity. By accident, too, I came across some description of the somatic and psychologic accompaniments of catatonic stupor, and decided, there and then, that the effect of drugs on this syndrome might be of interest. At that time, Jean Delay came over to London. It was his first contact across the Channel since the war; and he told us of his experiments of the effects of Amytal in catatonic stupor. (I was not aware of Lindemann's work [22] at that time.) Shorvon was developing his ether abreactive techniques.[23] We decided to embark on a study and to look for clinical material at the local mental hospital. I obtained a small grant for this work from the hospital research fund, and advertised for a research associate. No response was forthcoming; but one evening, when I was despondently telling Charmian, my wife, who was in general practice at the time, about the lack of appeal for a job of this kind, another of those incredible taps of fate took place. For quietly and unexpectedly, she asked me whether I had thought of her in this context. I said that I honestly hadn't, but was delighted at her interest, and immediately started gushing at her about the opportunities the job offered. Now, nothing gets my wife's back up more than extravagance and enthusiasm. She resisted; she considered it, and weighed it very carefully, finally deciding that she would give it a try.

We began to work at once at the Winson Green Mental Hospital (The Birmingham City Mental Hospital), whose Superintendent, J. J. O'Reilly, proved a real friend. He put a small research room at our disposal, allowed us to choose our patients from the rich population according to our criteria, and gave us nursing help. Thus our catatonia study developed with homemade gadgetry (to measure muscle "tone" and foot temperatures), which worked; with our own rating scales, which worked; with our own personal involvement, which taught both Charmian and me the enormous value of working in a realistic mental hospital setting. We communicated the results first to the Pharmacological Society of Great Britain, and then to psychiatric groups.[24, 25, 39a] They created a good deal of attention because of the well-known dramatic effects of Amytal, the paradoxical effects of amphetamine, the purely musculoskeletal effects of mephenesin, and the positive correlation of the psychomotor effect with peripheral vascular effects. The effects of the drugs on patients' drawings were also very striking.[25] Most important, however, these experiments established at a tangible "work" level, as well as at a conceptual level, the need of working in parallel at the bench and in the ward.

It was then, I suppose, that I decided that experimental psychiatry was clinical, or that it was nothing. Let it draw on the bench sciences, let it look for neural correlates of behavioral events in the animal model, let it delve as deeply as it can into processes governing the chemically mediated organ of information that we carry in our skull; but unless this yield from the bench is clearly and constantly related to the uniquely human events that are the business of psychiatry and of neuropsychology, the implications of such knowledge remain conjectural. All this is pretty obvious nowadays. In those days, however, in a Department of Pharmacology in Birmingham, it became part of a *plan.* I felt instinctively that the drugs we were working with, and the drugs that I was sure were coming (these were still the days before the discovery of LSD-25 and chlorpromazine) were tools of great precision and power, depending, one hoped, as in the case of the anticholinesterases, on one or two overriding properties. It is this kind of precision pharmacology of the central nervous system that made me hopeful and made me take up my stance in the face of raised eyebrows, which I encountered not only in the Physiological Society but also in psychiatric circles, where I was regarded as a maverick, newcomer and curiosity. I read the question, "What is the fellow up to?" on every face; although, it is possible that there was interest in this question also.

At that time, then, there were two anchoring points for my work in the mental disease field: neurochemistry, at the bench level, and human behavior, as influenced by drugs. There was nothing in between, no indicator to relate the effects of drugs on the brain in the conscious animal to behavior, nor any correlation between behavior and brain chemistry. I began to look and hunt again; the EEG was at that time coming into its own. Hill and Pond [26, 27] were publishing on the dysrhythmias, and Grey Walter [28] and Gastaut [29] were in their own idiom trying to relate functional states in man to EEG activity. And across the water there beckoned the great papers of Herbert Jasper [30]; and Wilder Penfield's finding electrified me.[31] I plumbed for the effect of drugs on the electrical activity of the brain in the conscious animal. There were very few data available in those days except those of Abraham Wikler [32] and James Toman's review.[33] I obviously could not do it alone, and again I was in the market for an associate.

I cannot recall now who told Philip Bradley about me or me about Philip Bradley; but I remember clearly his coming to my office and telling me of his experience and his interests. He had been trained in zoology, and had carried out microelectrode studies in insects. He seemed interested in the problem, and a salary was available. So, after some consultation with Dr. Grey Walter, arrangements were made for him to spend some time with Grey Walter, and then to set up his own laboratory in the second of the two rooms of "Mental Diseases Research." This was duly done; and in 1947 or '48, Philip was working alongside, developing his pioneering technique for recording the electrical activity in the conscious animal,[34] a procedure that in those days (before penicillin in England) was quite a trick. The work proceeded well, and quickly established reference points for the pharmacology of the brain, inasmuch as it relates to behavior. It was a joy to see the clear and unambiguous effects of physostigmine, atropine, hyoscyamine, and amphetamine (and later, LSD-25) on the electrical activity of the brain in relation to behavior.[34-36] It was also particularly satisfying to find how these drugs grouped themselves in terms of their dependence on midbrain structures, how information arriving at that time from Moruzzi and Magoun's studies [37] could be related to our own findings, and how the whole complex of the emerging "reticular formation" (which has since been fractionated much more discretely) fitted our data. There gradually emerged (and this was my own view) a concept of the presence of *families* of compounds that had arisen in the brain, in the course of chemical evolution, and that were chemically related to powerful neurohumoral transmitters familiar to us at the periphery.[24,36,39] Three types of receptors, centering around members of the cholinester, the catecholamine and, later, the indole family, were proposed. Implicit in this concept of families of compounds were the concepts of small, local chemical fields; and of the interaction and interdependence between such molecules in governing, modulating and gating storage and flow in self-exciting neural loops. Reciprocal inhibition was regarded as the agent of structure in the central nervous system. I have modified these ideas somewhat since, and expressed them in various papers [38-40]; but the concept of families of compounds, derived and evolved from respective common chemical roots, governing the physiology of the brain (and, by implication, the chemistry of awareness, perception, affect and memory) was a steady part of my thinking as we worked away in Birmingham; and, to the best of my knowledge, represents the first formulation of these ideas.

Two other events influenced my future course of action. In 1949, I had a severe attack of influenza. I lay in bed and was catching up on my technical reading. One report was the review by Mark Nickerson on adrenergic blockade [41]; and mentioned in it, tucked away among the ergonovine derivatives was a paragraph referring to Stoll's [42] since-famous paper describing the properties of a lysergic acid derivative, LSD-25. I was galvanized by the dose level here mentioned—10 to 30 μmg by mouth, and immediately began to think in terms of mode of action. I wrote to the local representative of Messrs. Sandoz and obtained, in a sealed tube, a small sample of LSD-25, which Bradley and I proceeded to use in our cat experiments. As far as I know, this was one of the first, if not the first sample of the material in use in a laboratory in Great Britain. However, we did not use it in man until 1951, after I had come back from a year in the United States. The experiments in the cat showed the effect of LSD-25 on the corticogram, both spontaneous and following rhythmic photic stimulation; the exquisite dependence of a response on the precise environmental setting, and its dependence on afferent input. It was an extraordinarily exciting time. Bradley and I reported on the effects of amphetamine and LSD-25 at the January, 1953, meeting of the Physiological Society [43]; and at the April, 1953, meeting, Gaddum reported his now classic observation of the antagonism of LSD-25 and serotonin.[44] All our experimental facts became relevant in proposing later [45] that the LSD-sensitive receptor might be peculiarly related to the afferent system (possibly to the medial afferent collaterals) and exercise a selective inhibitory role in the organization of sensory information—a proposal not out of keeping with Aghajanian's recent findings.[45a-46]

As I said, the human experiment did not follow until 1951, when I took the first dose of LSD-25 in the presence of Bradley and my wife, as part of an experiment that was to involve 15 volunteers. I remember the day, two days before Christmas. The sheer physical setting of the experiment was horrendous. We had no human experimental laboratory of any kind; so we cleared out the cat cages and cat observation box in Philip Bradley's laboratory, put a mattress on the bench in a dark room, with the EEG leads coming out of a small window behind, and let the drug take its course. We had only one paper to guide us. Our subjects were chosen on the basis of availability and interest.

The personal experience was intense and exquisite, and gave one an insight never to be forgotten of the full, mysterious sensation that one might describe as the antechambers of the full psychedelic experience. Mainly, this experiment explored subjective effects in subjects of very different make-up; the effects of reduction of sensory input in a dark room, while the EEG was being taken; the effects on the spontaneous EEG; the effects on EEG following stroboscopic stimulation at different frequencies; the effect of environment and anticipation, set and setting. All this was taken up later in other laboratories.

Here is the abstract of our communication [45]:

> LSD 25 (Stoll, 1947) was administered by mouth in doses of 15-100 μg to twelve male and three female volunteers, and particular attention was paid to the effects of rhythmic photic stimulation (effected by an electronic stroboscope at 4-24 c/s) on the symptoms of intoxication. The subjective sensations, including the illusions of form, colour and movement experienced under these conditions, were sound-recorded for each frequency. An EEG record was then taken and photic stimulation repeated during the recording. The drug was then administered. Symptoms generally appeared within 20-30 min and with three exceptions, were quite apparent within the hour. The stroboscope run was then repeated, first without, then with, the EEG electrodes in place. As before, all verbal material was recorded.
>
> Broadly the symptoms observed were those described by Stoll; depersonalization, heightened awareness, and fluctuating, incongruous affect were the most common symptoms. Eight subjects experienced visual symptoms, and seven distortion of body image. Mild dysarthria was seen in eleven, and thought blocking in six subjects. Rhythmic photic stimulation enhanced the symptoms in twelve out of fifteen subjects, and in three out of these twelve, symptoms were brought out where no symptoms of any kind had been experienced before. An incommunicative trance-like state during photic stimulation following LSD 25 was experienced by six subjects; and in three there was a slight, transient but quite definite alteration in muscle tone (not unlike that seen in catatonia), which persisted for up to 20 min after photic stimulation had ceased. . . .

Particularly, what should be noted is the "trance-like" state induced in some. Three of our subjects showed visual and affective after effects lasting for months after the experiment. One experienced what, these days, would be described as a very bad "trip," despite a moderate dose. In those days the only antidote available to us was Amytal Sodium.

While we were engaged in these experiments, Drs. Sandison and Spencer, colleagues in Birmingham and working in Powick Mental Hospital, some miles away, began their pioneering studies of the use of LSD-25 as a treatment of malignant obsessional and related states.[47] One dark afternoon, our local little research society was to meet at Powick Hospital. The weather was foul, and only five of us turned up at the meeting. But I still remember the astonishment with which I listened to Dr. Sandison's paper on the therapeutic effects of LSD-25 and, particularly, the rich symbolic material with which he illustrated his paper. I had a feeling that I had listened to something important: Between our own work and the work of others, the world of the psychodysleptics was opening up wide.

The other clinical trial concerned the advent of chlorpromazine. We were at that time deeply impressed by Charmian's finding of the paradoxical effects of Amytal, amphetamine, mephenesin and, later, LSD-25 in catatonic schizophrenic stupor.[25] We also were taken with the findings of Hill, Pond and others suggesting temporal lobe dysfunction in aggressive antisocial states,[26, 27] and possibly in schizophrenia. We were wondering whether the so-called anti-epileptic drugs had a place in the treatment of these disorders, and were about to organize a trial of diphenylhydantoin; but then one day there walked into my office Dr. W. R. Thrower, of Messrs. May and Baker. He said it was not a routine visit. He showed me a report in English translation of the findings of Delay and Deniker concerning chlorpromazine, a draft of their classic paper.[48] Dr. Thrower told me that May and Baker had acquired the British rights for chlorpromazine. Would we care to carry out the trial? Being very impressed by Delay and Deniker's report, I said we certainly would like to, and that we could do so at Winson Green Mental Hospital. I asked Charmian whether she would be interested; she said she would, and assumed full responsibility for the management of what was to prove, I think, a rather important step in clinical psychopharmacology. For, as I think back on it, all the difficulties, all the opportunities, all the unpredictable qualities of conducting a trial in a mental hospital setting were to show up clearly, and to be dealt with clearly, in that very early trial: the preparation of the ward, the training of personnel, the gullibility of us all—the so-called "halo" effect when faced with a novel situation—the cooperation on the part of the medical and nonmedical personnel, the importance of nursing attendants, relatives and patients themselves as informants; the use of rating scales and the calibration of such scales—all these elements came into their own, once Charmian, and to a much lesser extent I, were faced with the realities of the trial. Our short paper, which conclusively proved the value of chlorpromazine,[49] and was the subject of an editorial in *The British Medical Journal,* was a blind self-controlled trial of chlorpromazine. But it was more; for it was a statement of the opportunities offered by a mental hospital for work of this kind, the difficulties one was likely to encounter, and the rules that one had to observe to obtain results. As we wrote:

> Perhaps we may be allowed to draw attention to one last point—namely, the lessons we feel we have learnt from the trial itself. The research instrument in a trial of this sort being a group of people, and its conduct being inseparable from the individual use of words, we were impressed by the necessity for a 'blind' and self-controlled design and independent multiple documentation. Furthermore, we were equally impressed by the false picture apt to be conveyed if undue reliance was placed on interview alone, as conducted in the clinic room. The patients' behavior in the ward was apt to be very different. For that reason the day and night nursing staff became indispensable and valued members of the observers' team. We were warmed and encouraged by the energy and care with which they did what was requested of them, provided this was clearly and simply set out at the beginning. A chronic 'back' ward thus became a rather interesting place to work in. There may well be a case for training senior nursing staff in elementary research method and in medical documentation. This would make for increased interest, increased attention to, and respect for detail, and the availability of a fund of information, all too often lost because it has not been asked for.[49]

Both these trials took place in a department that by that time I had been invited to found—by the new Dean of the Medical School, Professor, later Sir Arthur, Thomson: the Department of Experimental Psychiatry, the University of Birmingham. As indicated, the laboratory facilities were readily available and had grown out of my previous experience. But, as I said earlier, psychiatry—even experimental psychiatry—is clinical or it is nothing. When we constructed our department, we decided clearly, and early, that it was to have a clinical arm as well as an experimental arm. The laboratories were in the school of medicine, in a small new building provided by the Hospital Board. At the same time, a clinical setting was founded, both in the City Mental Hospital and in a special clinic created at the time with the help of William Mayer-Gross, who joined me as a principal clinical associate in 1955. The Uffculme Clinic, as it was called, comprised some 40 beds, a day hospital, and an active outpatient clinic. There were also biochemical laboratories and ethology laboratories led by Dr. Michael Chance; I believe this was the first ethology laboratory to be established in a department of psychiatry. The Rockefeller Foundation gave us most generous support. So did the Medical Research Council of Great Britain. I am glad to say that to this day this Clinic is functioning very well, and is now a main teaching center of the Birmingham Regional Hospital complex centered around the Birmingham University School of Medicine. After my departure for the United States in 1957, my department was divided into a Department of Experimental Neuropharmacology, under Professor Philip Bradley, and a Clinical Department of Psychiatry, under Professor William Trethowan, now Dean of the Medical Faculty. Graduate teaching continues.

NEUROPHARMACOLOGY AND PSYCHOPHARMACOLOGY IN WASHINGTON, DC

As I mentioned earlier, I had spent a year (1950-1951) in the United States, having had the good fortune to have awarded to me the first Smith, Kline, and French Traveling Fellowship, awarded to me in England, and to get a Fulbright Award. I had a stimulating time at the late Dr. Samuel Wortis' Institute at New York University, visiting also Dr. Fritz Redlich's Institute at Yale, and also working very productively at the Pratt Diagnostic Center at Boston with Dr. John Nemiah, who taught me much. One of the most poignant experiences, however, was again to come by way of the pull of a mental hospital. Somehow, I felt that an enormous treasury of natural history of disease was lying there; and when I met with Dr. Redlich, I asked him whether it would not be advisable for me to get to know an American state hospital at first hand.

It was duly arranged that I should spend five months at Norwich State Hospital, Connecticut. This was done through the courtesy of the late Dr. Kettle, Superintendent of the Hospital, a wonderful person to work with and for. At that time, too, we discussed the question of building a research center at Norwich State Hospital; and it was some 10 years later that I got a joyous letter from Dr. Kettle that he had obtained funds to create such a Center, which, now, is the Abraham Ribicoff Center for Mental Health Research at Norwich State Hospital.

It is strange to reflect how constant are the constants of one's life, for when, in 1957, I received an invitation from the National Institutes of Health to create the Clinical Neuropharmacology Research Center of that Institute, I again favored a mental hospital (St. Elizabeths in Washington, DC) as a setting. With Dr. Robert Felix's strong and constant support, with the devoted help, enthusiasm and exceptional understanding of Drs. Robert Cohen and Seymour Kety, we established the Clinical Neuropharmacology Research Center at the William A. White Building of the hospital. I will not hide the fact that it was hard going at first. We started, in 1957, with a secretary (Mrs. Anne Gibson) and myself in a large dark, "Continued Care" building containing some 300 patients. But staff came —Drs. Neil Waldrop, Hans Weil-Malherbe, G. C. Salmoiraghi, Shepherd Kellam, S. Szara, Hordern, Lofft, Max Hamilton, Eliot Hearst and Harold Weiner, Richard Michael and many others. The laboratories and research Wards of the Center grew and grew. In 1961, Fritz Freyhan joined the Center as Director of Clinical Studies.

Again, some of the same themes (in variation) reappeared, though I cannot mention them all: microelectrophysiology, which, in Dr. Salmoiraghi's hands, became a pioneering technique for the study of the pharmacology of single neurons in the central nervous system [50]; amine metabolism, under Dr. Weil-Malherbe [51]; the metabolism of psychodysleptic tryptamine derivates, under Dr. Szara [52]; animal behavioral studies, combining Skinnerian avoidance training with metabolic experiments under Dr. Hearst [53]; the effect of locally and isotopically labeled implanted hormones on behavior, under Dr. Richard Michael [54]; human behavior analysis studies under Dr. Harold Weiner [55]; the methodology of clinical drug trials under Drs. Hordern and Lofft [56]; the quantification of social interaction in a psychiatric ward under Dr. Shepherd Kellam [57]; and the conceptualization of comprehensive mental health care in a given community by Dr. Freyhan.[58] With the help of the late Dr. Winfred Overholser, Superintendent of St. Elizabeths Hospital, the Behavioral and Clinical Studies Center of St. Elizabeths was created as a complementary entity.

I am glad to say that this enterprise is doing nicely, too, at present. In the last three years, particularly, the whole program, now the Division of Special Mental Health Programs of the National Institute of Mental Health, has assumed dynamic leadership under Dr. G. C. Salmoiraghi, and greatly expanded its scope, with the joining of Dr. Costa, Dr. Bloom, Dr. McDonald, Dr. Veitch, and others. It is now a world resource in the field of neuropsychopharamacology.

Though I have been at Johns Hopkins since 1963, my former colleagues and I still maintain contact. The handsomely bound Collection of their Reprints, which they gave me when I left in 1963, is the nicest present I ever had. At Johns Hopkins there is much else to do besides psychopharmacology; but we have the good fortune of a convergence of interests in theoretical and applied Psychopharmacology through my colleagues Dr. Solomon Snyder (Psychiatry and Neurochemistry), Dr. Joseph Brady and Dr. Jack Findley (Behavior Analysis) and Drs. Joseph Stephens, L. Faillace, Lino Covi, and Herbert Weingartner (Clinical Studies). Keen new students continue to press into the field every year. Our interests center on the mode of action of some amphetamine analogs and hallucinogens, on the relation of dopamine storage to the mode of action of antiparkinson agents, and the intriguing properties of an old friend, diphenylhydantoin.

THE EMERGENCE OF ORGANIZATIONS

Looking back, in 1970, with large national and international organizations in psychopharmacology spanning the globe, and vast industrial undertakings engaged in research, development and manufacture, it is a little hard to visualize the sparse and intimate nature of our field a mere eighteen years ago. I remember sitting in Heinrich Waelsch's study, overlooking the Hudson, in August 1951, just before returning to England to take up the newly created post of Head of the Department of Experimental Psychiatry. "What *is* experimental psychiatry?" asked Heinrich Waelsch, giving me that whimsical penetrating look of his. The newly created Professor did not rightly know. "I suppose," I said, hesitatingly "it is the application of experimental research method to clinical psychiatry; I suppose, in my own case, it is the application of chemistry to an analysis and understanding of behavior. I will tell you when I have done it for a while."

Later, back in England, I got in touch with Drs. Derek Richter and Geoffrey Harris; Heinrich Waelsch met with Drs. Seymour Kety, Jordi Folch-Pi, and Louis Flexner. Our joint hope, which we had shared at a previous small meeting, was to organize an International Neurochemical Symposium, the first of its kind. As the theme of the symposium, we significantly chose "The Biochemistry of the Developing Nervous System." As a place to hold it, we chose Magdalen College, Oxford. I was charged with being organizing Secretary, but could not have done it without the devoted help of my British colleagues. Sixty-nine colleagues from nine countries participated. It was a fine symposium; the conversation was good and ranged wide. It may be that it was at this symposium that the term *neurochemistry* was used officially for the first time. The spirit of the meeting is perhaps conveyed in an extract from the Preface that Heinrich Waelsch and I wrote for the Proceedings[59]:

> We agreed also that from the start it would be well to consider the brain as a biological entity in all its complexity of morphology and function, rather than as a homogenate, or an engineering problem. For that reason, we felt that the most useful contribution of a Symposium of this kind would be an attempt to reintegrate biochemical process with structure and function, particularly with respect to the chemical topography of the brain, which, to us, seemed of greatest moment in an understanding of function. The program thus not only represents the framework of a conference, but also expresses an attitude; and of necessity includes discussion of structural, genetic, and pathological aspects, as well as subject matter that in the more limited sense may be termed "neurochemical." We feel that this approach may be helpful in slowly building the foundations for a rational therapy of disorders of the nervous system.

These international symposia have continued, the fourth held, in 1960, being devoted to regional neurochemistry,[60] a topic very much with us today.

In the meantime, other important events were stirring. The Macy Symposia on Neuropharmacology, initiated by Dr. Harold Abramson in 1954,[61] brought a number of us together; and in 1956, under the joint chairmanship of Drs. Jonathan Cole and Ralph Gerard, a milestone Conference on Psychopharmacology was held under the aegis of the National Research Council, and the National Academy of Science and the American Psychiatric Association [62]: during which year, also, Dr. Cole's Psychopharmacology Service Center was created, a step of enormous consequences for the future development of the field all over the world.

In 1957, the World Health Organization invited me to serve as consultant, and convened a small Study Group on the subject of Ataractic and Hallucinogenic Drugs in Psychiatry. The following participated:

Dr. Ludwig von Bertalanffy (USA)
Dr. U. S. von Euler (Sweden)
Dr. E. Jacobsen (Denmark)
Dr. Morton Kramer (USA)
Dr. T. A. Lambo (Nigeria)
Dr. E. Lindemann (USA)
Dr. P. Pichot (France)
Dr. D. McK. Rioch (USA)
Dr. R. A. Sandison (England)
Dr. P. B. Schneider (Switzerland)

I wrote the report,[63] which, incidentally, carried Eric Jacobsen's pioneer classification of the main drugs according to their pharmacological properties. In the meantime, the Scientific Command of the US Air Force, through its principal representative in Europe, Col. James Henry, had catalyzed important work in the neurological sciences in a number of European laboratories. Through these meetings, the international implications of brain research became steadily more apparent. After preliminary meetings in 1958, 1959, and 1960, a number of us met in UNESCO House in 1960 to draft the statutes and by-laws of IBRO—the International Brain Research Organization. The disciplines of neuroanatomy, neurochemistry, neuroendocrinology, neuropharmacology, neurophysiology, behavioral sciences, neurocommunications and biophysics were represented. Dr. Daniel Bovet and I represented neuropharmacology on the Central Council of IBRO.

At about the same time, national groups in psychopharmacology began to form, at first loosely and informally, and later in more definitive ways. That most important international body, the Collegium Internationale Neuropsychopharmacologicum was born in 1957; and, reflecting Drs. E. Rothlin's and Abraham Wikler's energy and devotion, our own journal of psychopharmacology—*Psycho-*

pharmacologia, representing our own new science, saw the light of day in 1959, and has continued as a yardstick of excellence since.

There are many other memories that flood the mind, but clearly these reminiscences have gone on much too long, and I must bring them to a close. When the American College of Neuropsychopharmacology was constituted in Washington in 1960, and did me the immense honor of electing me their first president, I could not help remembering that this had happened only 15 years after I had played with macromolecular models and the x-ray diffraction of myelin in my laboratory in Birmingham, and only 10 years after we had created a Department of Experimental Psychiatry in Birmingham. I could not help reflecting on the unique power of our field to act not only as a catalyst but as a binder; a catalyst bringing into being whole new areas of science, but also as a binder and a relator of these sciences to each other. For we had not only to create fields of investigation and measuring devices in many disciplines, but also a degree of understanding and interaction between disciplines, which is very rare. As I said at the time,

> It is not uncommon for any one of us to be told that Psychopharmacology is not a science, and that it would do well to emulate the precision of older and more established disciplines. Such statements betray a lack of understanding for the special demands made by Psychopharmacology upon the fields which compound it. For my own part, I draw comfort and firm conviction from the history of our subject, and the history of our group. For I know of no other branch of science which, like a good plough on a spring day, has tilled as many areas in Neurobiology. To have, in a mere decade, questioned the concepts of synaptic transmission in the central nervous system; to have emphasized compartmentalization and regionalization of chemical process in the unit cell and in the brain; to have focussed on the interaction of hormone and chemical process within the brain; to have given us tools for the study of the chemical basis of learning and temporary connection formation; to have emphasized the dependence of pharmacological response on its situational and social setting; to have compelled a hard look at the semantics of psychiatric diagnosis, description and communication; to have resuscitated that oldest of old remedies, the placebo response, for careful scrutiny; to have provided potential methods for the study of language in relation to the function state of the brain; and to have encouraged the Biochemist, Physiologist, Psychologist, Clinician, and the Mathematician and Communication Engineer to join forces at bench level, is no mean achievement for

a young science. That a chemical text should carry the imprint of experience, and partake in its growth, in no way invalidates study of symbols, and the rules among symbols, which keep us going, changing, evolving, and human.

Thus, though moving cautiously, psychopharmacology is still protesting; yet, in so doing it is, for the first time, compelling the physical and chemical sciences to look behavior in the face, and thus enriching both these sciences and behavior. If there be discomfiture in this encounter, it is hardly surprising; for it is in this discomfiture that there may well lie the germ of a new science.

In our branch of science, it would seem we are as attracted to substance as we are to symbol; we are as interested in behavior as we are aware of the subleties of subjective experience. There is here no conflict between understanding the way things are, and the way people are, between the pursuit of science and the giving of service.

Where else does one find a field as rich and powerful as ours?

REFERENCES

1. Elkes, J., Frazer, A. C., and Stewart, H. C.: The composition of particles seen in normal human blood under ground illumination, J Physiol (London) *95:*68, 1939.

2. Schmitt, Francis O.: X-ray diffraction studies on nerve, Radiology *25:* 131, 1935.

3. ——: X-ray diffraction studies on structure of nerve myelin sheath, J Cell Physiol *18:*31, 1941.

4. Elkes, J., and Finean, J. B.: The effect of drying upon the structure of myelin in the sciatic nerve of the frog, *in* Discussion of the Faraday Society, Lipoproteins, 1949, p. 134.

5. ——: X-ray diffraction studies on the effect of temperature on the structure of myelin in the sciatic nerve of the frog, Exp Cell Res *4:*69 ,1953.

6. ——: Effects of solvents on the structure of myelin in the sciatic nerve of the frog, *ibid.*, p. 82.

7. Richter, Derek: Metabolism of the Nervous System, New York, Pergamon, 1957.

8. Austin, J. H.: *In* Bogoch, S., ed.: The Future of the Brain Sciences, New York, Plenum, 1969. p. 403.

9. Finean, James B.: Chemical Ultrastructure in Living Tissues, Springfield (Ill), Thomas, 1961.

10. Engstrom, A., and Finean, J. B.: Biological Ultrastructure, New York, Acad Press, 1958.

11. Elkes, J., and Todrick, A.: On the development of the cholinesterases in the rat brain, *in* Waelsch, H., ed.: Biochemistry of the Developing Nervous System, New York, Acad Press, 1955, p. 309.

12. Elkes, J., Eayrs, J. T., and Todrick, A.: On the effect and the lack of effect of some drugs on postnatal deveolpment in the rat, *ibid.*, p. 499.

13. Page, Irvine, H.: Chemistry of the Brain, Springfield (Ill), Thomas, 1937.

14. Michaelis, M., and Quastel, J. H.: Site of action of narcotics in respiratory processes, Biochem J *35:*518, 1941.

15. Himwich, H. E., Bowman, K. M., Fazekas, J. F., and Goldfarb, W.: Temperature and brain metabolism, Amer J Med Sci: *200*:347, 1940.

16. Richter, Derek: Inactivation of adrenaline *in vivo* in man, J Physiol (London) *98*:361, 1940.

17. Thudichum, John, W. L.: A Treatise on the Chemical Constitution of the Brain, London, Balliere, 1884.

18. Masserman, Jules, H.: An analysis of the influence of alcohol on experimental neuroses in cats, Psychosom Med *8*:36, 1946.

19. McDougall, William: The Frontiers of Psychology, Cambridge (Eng), Univ Press, 1935.

20. Feldberg, W., and Vogt, M.: Acetylcholine synthesis in different regions of central nervous system, J Physiol (London) *107*:372, 1948.

21. Kluver, H.: Mechanisms of hallucinations, *in* McNemar, Q., and Merrill, M. A., eds: Studies in Personality, New York, McGraw-Hill, 1942, p. 175.

22. Lindemann, Erich, and Malamud, William: Experimental analysis of the psychopathological effects of intoxicating drugs, Amer J Psychiat *13*:853, 1934.

23. Sargant, W., and Shorvon, H. J.: Acute war neuroses, Arch Neurol (Chicago) *54*:231, 1945.

24. Elkes, J., Elkes, C., and Bradley, P. B.: The effect of some drugs on the electrical activity of the brain and on behavior, J Ment Sci *100*:125, 1954.

25. Elkes, J.: Some effects of psychosomimetic drugs on the experimental animal, and in man, *in:* Neuropharmacology, Transactions of the Third Conf, Josiah Macy, Jr., Foundation, 1957, pp. 205-294.

26. Hill, D.: Cerebral dysrhythmia: its significance in aggressive behavior, Proc Roy Soc Med *37*:317, 1944.

27. Hill, D., and Pond, D. A.: Reflections on one hundred capital cases submitted to electroencephalography, J Ment Sci *98*:23, 1952.

28. Walter, V. J., and Walter, W. G.: The central effects of rhythmic sensory stimulation, Electroenceph Clin Neurophysiol *1*:57, 1949.

29. Gastaut, H.: Combined photic and metrazol activation of the brain, Electroenceph Clin Neurophysiol *2*:263, 1950.

30. Jasper, H.: Symposium: thalamocortical relationships; diffuse projection systems: integrative action of thalamic reticular system, Electroenceph Clin Neurophysiol *1*:405, 1949.

31. Penfield, Wilder: Ferrier Lecture: Some observations on cerebral cortex of man, Proc Roy Soc Med *134*:329, 1947.

32. Wikler, A.: Pharmacologic dissociation of behavior and EEG 'sleep patterns' in dogs; morphine, n-allylnormorphine and atrophine, Proc Soc Exp Biol Med *79*:261, 1952.

33. Toman, James: Pharmacol Rev *1*:425, 1949.

34. Elkes, Joel, and Bradley, P. B.: A technique for recording the electrical activity of the brain in the conscious animal, Electroenceph Clin Neurophysiol *5*:451, 1953.

35. Bradley, P. B., and Elkes, J.: The effect of atropine, hyoscyamine physostigmine and neostigmine on the electrical activity of the brain of the conscious cat, J Physiol (London) *120*:14, 1953.

36. ——: The effects of some drugs on the electrical activity of the brain, Brain *80*:77, 1957.

37. Moruzzi, G., and Magoun, H. W.: Brainstem reticular formation and activation of the EEG, Electroenceph Clin Neurophysiol *1*:455, 1949.

38. Elkes, J.: Drug effects in relation to receptor specificity within the brain: some evidence and provisional formulation, Ciba Foundation Symposium on the Neurological Basis of Behavior, 1958, p. 303.

39. ——: Drugs influencing affect and behavior: possible neural correlates in relation to mode of action, *in* Simon, A., ed.: The Physiology of Emotions, Springfield (Ill), Thomas, 1961, p. 95.

39a. ——: *In* Tanner, J. M., ed.: Prospects in Psychiatric Research, Oxford (Eng), Blackwell, 1953, p. 126.

40a. ——: Psychoactive drugs: Some problems and approaches, *in* Solomon, Philip, ed.: Psychiatric Drugs, New York, Grune, 1966, pp. 4-21.

40b. ——: Behavioral pharmacology in relation to psychiatry, *in* Psychiatric der Gegenwart, Heidelberg, Springer, 1967, pp. 931-1038.

41. Nickerson, Mark: The pharmacology of adrenergic blockade, Pharmacol Rev *1:*27, 1949.

42. Stoll, A.: Lysergsaure-diathylamid, ein Phantastikum aus der Mutterkorngruppe, Schweiz Arch Neurol Neurochir Psychiat *60:*279, 1947.

43. Bradley, P. B., and Elkes, J.: The effect of amphetamine and d-lysergic acid diethylamide (LSD-25) on the electrical activity of the brain of the conscious cat, J Physiol (London) *120:*13, 1953.

44. Gaddum, J. H.: Antagonism between lysergic acid diethylamide and 5-hydroxytryptamine, J Physiol (London) *121:*15, 1953.

45. Elkes, J.: *Op. cit.*, ref. 38, pp. 327-328.

45a. Aghajanian, G. K.: Effects of LSD on raphe nuclei neurons Neurosciences Res Program Bull *8:*40-54, 1970.

46. Bradley, P. B., Elkes, C., and Elkes, J.: On some effects of lysergic acid diethylamide (LSD-25) in normal volunteers, J Physiol (London) *121:*50, 1953.

47. Sandison, R. A., Spencer, A. M., and Whitelaw, J. D. A.: J Ment Sci *100:*491, 1954.

48. Delay, J., and Deniker, P.: Les neuroplegiques en therapeutique psychiatrique, Thérapie *8:*347, 1953.

49. Elkes, J., and Elkes, C.: Effects of chlorpromazine on the behavior of chronically overactive psychotic patients, Brit Med J *2:*560, 1954.

50. Salmoiraghi, G. C., and Bloom, F. E.: Pharmacology of individual neurons, Science *144:*493, 1964.

51. Weil-Malherbe, H., Posner, H., and Bowles, G.: Changes in the concentration and intracellular distribution on brain catecholamines: the effects of reserpine, β-phenylisoprophylhydrazine, pyrogallol and 3-4-dihydroxyphenylalanine alone and in combination, J Pharmacol Exp Ther *132:*278, 1961.

52. Szara, S., Hearst, E., and Putney, F.: Metabolism in behavioral action of psychotropic tryptamine homologues, Int J Neuropharmacol *1:*111, 1962.

53. Szara, S., and Hearst, E.: The 6 hydroxylation of tryptamine derivatives: a way of producing psychoactive metabolites, Ann NY Acad Sci *96:*134, 1962.

54. Michael, R. P.: An investigation of the sensitivity of circumscribed neurological areas to hormonal stimulation by means of the application of oestrogens directly to the brain of the cat, *in* Kety, S., and Elkes, J., eds.: Regional Neurochemistry, Oxford (Eng), Pergamon, 1961, p. 465.

55. Weiner, Harold: Some effects of response cost upon human operant behavior J Exp Anal Behav *5:*201, 1962.

56. Hordern, Anthony, Hamilton, M., Waldrop, F. N., and Lofft, J. C.: A controlled trial on the value of prochlorperazine and trifluoperazine and intensive group treatment, Brit J Psychiat *109:*510-522, 1963.

57. Kellam, Sheppard G.: A method for assessing social contact: its application during a rehabilitation program on a psychiatric ward, J Nerv Ment Dis *132:*277, 1961.

58. Freyhan, F., and Mayo, J. A.: Concept of a model psychiatric clinic, Amer J Psychiat *120:*222, 1963.

59. Waelsch, Heinrich, ed.: Biochemistry of the Developing Nervous System, New York, Acad Press, 1955, p. 5.

60. Kety, S., and Elkes, J., eds.: Regional Neurochemistry, Proc 4th Int Neurochemical Symp, New York, Pergamon, 1961.

61. Abramson, Harold A., ed.: Neuropharmacology, New York, Josiah Macy, Jr., Foundation, 1954.

62. Cole, J. O., and Gerard, R. W., eds.: Psychopharmacology: Problems in Evaluation, Nat Acad Sci and Nat Res Council, Washington (DC), 1959.

63. WHO: Ataractic and Hallucinogenic Drugs in Psychiatry, World Health Organization Tech Rep Series No. 152, Geneva, 1958.

64. Elkes, J.: The American College of Neuropsychopharmacology: A Note on Its History, and Hopes for the Future, Amer Coll of Neuropsychopharmacology Bull *1:*(No. 1)2, 1963.

CHAPTER

3

Neurochemistry As I Have Known It

SEROTONIN

IRVINE H. PAGE, MD*

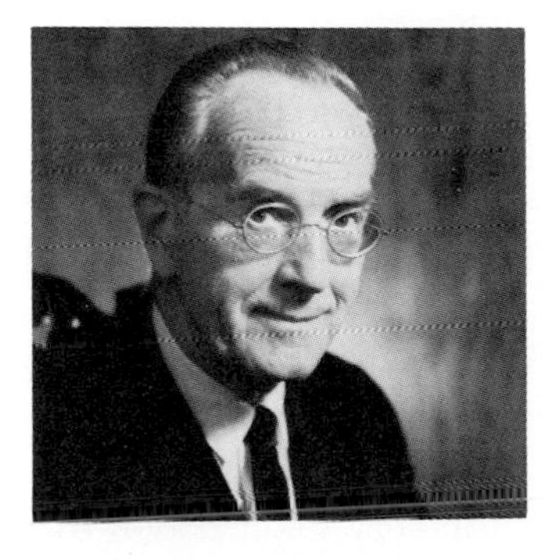

IN AUGUST, 1928, I set sail for Munich, Germany, to start a department of "brain chemistry" at the Kaiser Wilhelm Institute for psychiatry, also known as the "Kraepelin Institute." I had just finished my hospital training in New York and had intended to enter private practice. I wish I could tell you that my life has consisted of a series of carefully reasoned moves, based on foresight and good judgment—but the only one I recall was my marriage. The rest were the operations of fate, collaborating with a moderately dissident, odd fellow, who first thought he wanted to be a professional botanist, but was trained to be a professional chemist, and who, I suspect, might have boiled his draft card instead of burning it had he been young today.

"Brain—or neuro-chemistry" I had never heard of, and there was good reason that I shouldn't, for in 1928 there was none. It was not until two years later that I found that J. L. W. Thudichum in 1884 had written the first and *only* book on the subject, and then the whole business had been forgotten. There were those who thought the transmission of nerve impulses required no energy, and when

* Director emeritus, Research Division, The Cleveland Clinic Foundation, Cleveland.

my old friend, the professor of biochemistry at Cincinnati, A. P. Mathews, heard about my venture, he typically remarked: "Page as usual is flying under the black flag of piratism."

Quite simply, I liked the idea of having a paying job in Germany, especially Munich, where there were four resident Nobel Prize winners, three of whom became close friends, Richard Willstatter, Heinrich Wieland and Hans Fisher, and the fourth, Arnold Sommerfeld, I met. Any job would have suited me then, why not "brain chemistry?" As a result of exposure to German in grade school, I could fight a dragon but could not order a glass of beer.

I was invited to start the department, I am quite sure, by inadvertence. One day Dr. Walter Palmer, head of the medical service at the hospital in New York, called me to say that Geheimrat Willstatter wished me to attend his lecture that evening. He said that there must be some mistake, but why not go anyway! I did, and after the talk, the Geheimrat quite bluntly invited me to Munich. I accepted and that, ladies and gentlemen, is why I went into brain chemistry.

I found myself alone on the fourth floor of the psychiatric institute in bare rooms. Fortunately, Geheimrat Willstatter was to be my adviser and he gave me a free hand to equip it as I liked. When I compare what I did with a modern laboratory, I realize that I was a product of the old "separatory funnel" school of organic chemistry. The names given the various pieces of equipment, such as Thiele and Buchner, with which I had become familiar at Cornell, fortunately were the same in Munich for the very good reason that they had been invented there by many of the large staff of organic chemistry under Adolph von Baeyer, Willstatter's predecessor.

Our small group worked on what was then disparagingly called "schmier," which meant the lipids of the brain. Except for the industrial oil and fat chemists, the lipids had received little attention, even by the early biochemists. Remember at that time (1928), even cholesterol had no sure structure, and we added our bit by helping to show the correct position of the double bond, through our demonstration that cholestenone is alpha-beta-unsaturated ketone. We found the phospholipids to be made up of several kinds, many of which were later identified by Folch-Pi, who subsequently worked alongside me at the Rockefeller Institute. Since cholesterol esters had not been found in the brain, we thought perhaps enough of them had not been synthesized to make their properties clear;

so we prepared a whole series of them. Cholesterol had always been thought of as an extraordinarily stable building material and probably was not degraded. Remember the adrenal and sex hormones had not yet been discovered! We showed that breakdown probably occurred in the animal, though, of course, we were limited to balance experiments. We also found a possible intermediate in the form of cholestenone in arteriosclerotic aortas. When the work was published, neither paper created a ripple of interest, one reason being that what little was known suggested carbohydrate as the only metabolically active substance for brain. We characterized the lipids in Dercum's disease to see if diseases caused by the deposition of lipids like Hand-Schuller-Christian, Tay-Sachs or Gaucher's diseases were due to the material itself being abnormal or whether it simply could not be remobilized. As far as we could tell at that time, the deposits themselves in composition were not abnormal, suggesting an enzyme defect.

This must all seem very tame to the modern "molecular chemist," but then it helped in a small way to stimulate interest in cholesterol and other lipids. My interest in the sterols began when I separated an odd one from starfish eggs at the Marine Biological Laboratory in Woods Hole in 1918. I gave it what seemed to be a lovely name, "asteriasterol." Perhaps now that the starfish seems to be eating up the coral islands, people will get interested in the metabolism of these amazing creatures and their artificial parthenogenesis and leave Portnoy to his complaints. What I always liked about them was that you could cut off one part and a new one would grow, a procedure I would like to try on certain areas of myself!

During my stay in Germany, there were isolated studies in the general area but no recognized field of neurochemistry. Otto Loewi and Henry Dale had done their great work on acetylcholine. Quastel, Loebel, Gerard, Elliott, and Himwich were starting to measure respiration à la Warburg. The effects of irradiating ergosterol were discovered by Hess and Windaus. Berger described electrical brain waves. Rosenheim and Wieland were elucidating the structure of cholesterol and Levene the nature of nucleoproteins. Despite all these remarkable achievements, the field did not take form.

I say this advisedly because, in 1930, my army officer landlord told me that it would be most unwise to try to make my future in Germany. This advice he based on his intimate knowledge of the underground military group under General von Epp in Munich and the potential of Hitler who was in and out of Munich in those days. He convinced me that Germany was going to war and it would not be healthy for a foreigner to be there. But how to get back to the United States?

I wrote to many of my friends, but to get a job during the depression for an unknown in an outlandish business called "brain chemistry" seemed to them absurd. Neither neurologists nor psychiatrists thought that kind of work was needed. Those were the days when the clinician was king and a hybrid organic chemist-physician nothing at all. Apparently in 1930 I was one of the first "warmongers," if any of you remember this "accolade."

In discouragement, my wife and I decided it would be best to try for a job with whomever I really wanted most to work. There was no question in my mind that Dr. Donald Van Slyke was the man. I greatly admired his work but did not know him. One did not simply apply to the Rockefeller Institute; one waited to be asked. The problem was how to get asked. Two weeks later the telephone rang in the laboratory in Munich and a diffident voice identified the speaker as Dr. Van Slyke, calling from the Vierjahreszeiten Hotel. I couldn't believe it and was about to loose my usually uncivil tongue but something warned me! Van Slyke explained he had been told I was the only resident American physician, and would I look at his daughter's infected finger? The long and short of it was that no finger ever got better care, and I got invited to work with Van Slyke. I spent seven happy years with this magnificent man. I would love to talk about him but I must quit rambling. At any rate, this is why I became a cardiologist and have grown ancient in that field. The young call me "sir" and believe most of the stories I tell them come from an arteriosclerotic brain.

In 1937, my book *The Chemistry of the Brain* appeared and created hardly enough interest to be more than a publisher's remainder. The rest of the story of the florescence of neurochemistry is known to you because all of you provided the growth hormones. Surely, no more able and interesting men have ever been gathered together, for which we all owe a debt to Frank Ayd. Now the field has a journal, committees, international meetings, its household gods and traditions. Tradition of this sort reminds me a bit of a notice on the bulletin board of a young college, which said: "As of Monday morning, it will be traditional for freshmen to wear their caps on campus."

It was many years later, after the initial period of labeling myself a neurochemist (and finding myself wholly unsalable), that my attention unexpectedly returned. While working in Van Slyke's department in 1931, I was interested in blood-born vasoactive substances. I hoped some light might be shed on the mechanisms of hypertension. I was disturbed by the fact it was known that when blood clots, a vasoactive substance appears in serum. No one had any idea what it was, but if I expected to extract a substance present normally in the blood of hypertensives, I had to get rid of this interference. I continued work on it using the perfused rabbit's ear vessels after moving to the Indianapolis City Hospital in 1937. Despite the claim that the method was of little value, we found it reliable for rough quantitation and could characterize some of the properties of this intruder.

In 1945, Dr. Corcoran and I moved to the Cleveland Clinic and, with Dr. Arda Green and Maurice Rapport, isolated the pure substance and ultimately determined its structure as 5-hydroxytryptamine. We called it "serotonin." But strangely its interest turned out to be especially for the neurochemist! Dr. Betty Twarog, using the retractor muscle of *Mytilus* for assay, found serotonin in good quantity in the brain. I had come full circle. The story of serotonin is an interesting one because it seems to live a double life—one in the body and the other in the brain. Dr. McCubbin and I have called it "the amphibaric substance that has reestablished tenure for the pharmacologist." Serotonin illustrates the tenor of the times. Within a decade, thousands of papers have appeared on subjects ranging from its ability to antagonize LSD to being the cause of migraine headache and the dumping syndrome. But I must confess that the time sequences are now somewhat confused just as the note left by a housewife for the milkman: "Don't leave milk today. Of course, when I say today, I mean tomorrow, because I am writing this yesterday."

IN CONCLUSION

Brain chemistry has grown from a series of sporadic, disorganized efforts into an evolving discipline. It has still a long way to go until, as a specialty, it will wither away and die, because it will have become incorporated into a more general body of knowledge. The inquisitive can then traverse the circulatory canals with gun and camera, unimpeded by artificial borders defined by specialists. The body, like the world, must ultimately become one. The fact that there are so many of you who have already contributed so much in so short a time is testimony to my faith in what is ahead. Man will transmute this world and seek others to explore, but to do it he will need his one unique organ—the brain. Its chemical reactions must be in order; if they are not, the tools his imagination has already provided him will destroy him. It is only too probable that a missing or misplaced chemical group or a deformed molecule may unleash a force that will convert our bodies back to the elements. I am not so sure about the mind.

But if our molecular structure is in order, there can be no limits. I wonder when a minister says that the acids of science have rendered to tattered rags our faith in resurrection, immortality and the soul. Are these beliefs indeed merely wishful thinking, forever unsupportable by evidence? Is our limited span on earth our only life? As I come closer to my ancestors, I am even less sure because of the fleeting glimpses I have already had of the potentials of cerebral function.

Are we quite sure that mankind is not evolving into a higher state? Do we know whether psychic phenomena are assertions of the growing complexity of biological reality, and are spiritual phenomena also dependent upon biology? We who have dealt with the brain must be humbled by the ultimate question whether consciousness is an expression of neural complexity or an acknowledgment of the mystery of God.

This has been a discourse of one who originally thought of himself as a neurochemist and who turned out to be a cardiologist. I offer it for your attention because to me both science and medicine reflect people—those extraordinary animals who in some ways are more bestial than the beasts but in others seem destined to ultimate self-transcendence.

CHAPTER

4

Biological Psychiatric Treatments Preceding Pharmacotherapy

LOTHAR B. KALINOWSKY, MD, FAPA*

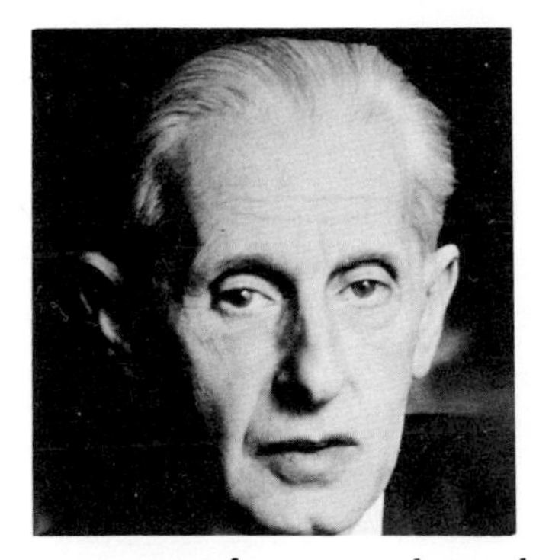

THE HISTORY OF EFFECTIVE BIOLOGICAL treatments in psychiatry is of such recent origin that it had its first beginnings during my own generation's professional life. By now, this field of endeavor has reached heights that none of us could dream of when we chose the specialty of psychiatry.

The first successful treatment for any mental illness was the malaria treatment for general paralysis introduced in Vienna by Wagner-von Jauregg in 1917. Like all subsequent biological treatments, malaria therapy had its origin in clinical observations made in mental hospitals. It had been seen frequently that certain psychotic patients improved dramatically during acute febrile diseases. After attempts with inoculation of recurrent fever, typhoid fever and other infections, malaria was chosen because, thanks to quinine, it was the best controllable infectious disease. Blood from humans containing malaria parasites was injected intramuscularly, and the patient allowed to have 10 or 12 fever bouts. It remained unclear whether the infection or the increased body temperature was responsible for the clinical improvement. Therefore, other heat-producing techniques like electrial lamps were also used. The beneficial effect of malaria therapy remained limited to patients with general paresis, and it was actually a way to immobilize and destroy spirochetes that

* Clinical Professor of Psychiatry, New York Medical College, New York.

had invaded the brain. Thus, malaria treatment cured a specific infection and was later replaced by penicillin; both these therapeutic means were not directed against the mental symptoms as such but against an underlying brain disease expressing itself in psychiatric manifestations.

Attempts to use malaria as well as other fever-producing methods in schizophrenia were made, among others, by Paul Hoch before he came to this country, but they remained unsuccessful. Still no treatment was available for any of the so-called functional psychoses like schizophrenia and manic-depressive psychosis. But the historical importance of malaria treatment of general paresis was that it ended the therapeutic nihilism of the generation of our great teachers who had given psychiatry its foundations but did not experiment with attempts at treatment.

This attitude began to change after the success of malaria therapy, and other therapeutic efforts were made. Thus, in 1922, the Swiss psychiatrist Klaesi introduced the so-called continuous sleep treatment, which can be considered the first modality of a somatic treatment used in the functional psychoses. The depth of the narcotic state induced by various hypnotics and the length of time during which patients were kept unconscious seemed to determine the beneficial effect. Acute excitement states of catatonic and manic patients responded best, but as a whole, results remained unsatisfactory. In some countries, like England and France, the treatment continued to have some clinical importance, and, with some technical deviations, was extensively used in the Soviet Union because it corresponded better than some other somatic treatments with certain concepts of Pavlovian psychiatry. In depressions, opium is another method used in the 1920's with unconvincing results.

It was my good fortune to become connected with the first biological method, namely, malaria treatment, in Hamburg, where a famous Institute for Tropical Diseases helped to establish the first German center for the use of malaria treatment of general paresis; and it was from here that I joined Wagner von Jauregg's staff and was assigned to Gerstmann and Dattner, his two co-workers in the development of malaria treatment. However, after a while, I went through an experience that still occurs today in the life of many young psychiatrists: It seemed much more sophisticated to concern oneself with the psychodynamics of psychopathological phenomena than with primitive physical treatments. I, therefore, switched to the psychoanalytical approach of Paul Schilder, who later became such a great influence on American psychiatry. However, Schilder's historical importance was that he was the first to recognize that psychological and biological concepts do not exclude each other. He determined the philosophy of Viennese psychiatry by showing equal interest in organic brain diseases and in psychopathology. It should be realized that most of the psychotherapeutic schools were well established at that time, when the biological treatment approach began to make its first strides that led to an unprecedented success story.

This story began with the introduction of "insulin shock treatment" by Sakel in 1933. This treatment—by means of hypoglycemic comas—was the first method directed at schizophrenia, the disease affecting the largest number of patients in all mental institutions. The discovery by Sakel, similar to the discovery of most subsequent biological treatments, was typical for the purely empirical and rather unscientific way all these newer treatment methods in psychiatry were found, a point that cannot be stressed enough and should keep our minds open for all clinical observations in our daily work if we want to find new clues in our search for newer and better treatments.

It was again the Psychiatric University Hospital in Vienna, under Wagner von Jauregg's successor Poetzl, that had a great influence on Sakel's introduction of insulin coma treatment, although Sakel began his work as the house physician in a small private sanitorium in my home town Berlin. Unknown to the Berlin University Hospital, where I worked at that time, he used insulin in a wide variety of psychiatric patients as it was then done for sedation and general build-up in many psychiatric hospitals and sanitoria. It was Sakel's brilliant idea to make clinical use of a phenomenon that other observers had also experienced but considered dangerous. Schizophrenic patients who happened to be hypersensitive to insulin and went into a hypoglycemic coma with unexpectedly low doses of insulin sometimes lost their psychotic symptomatology temporarily, subsequent to such an occurrence. This gave Sakel the courageous idea to produce hypoglycemic coma in schizophrenics at will.

In 1933, Sakel went to Vienna and, with the help of the excellent facilities of the therapeutically oriented University Hospital, established the technique of insulin coma treatment. This method, although wrongly neglected since the introduction of psychotropic drugs, was a turning point in psychiatry and brought our specialty closer to general medicine at a time when psychiatry still had not made any true progress in the understanding of the diseases with which it was dealing. Insulin "shock" treatment as Sakel called it, and the other so-called shock treatments that were to follow, soon altered the attitude of psychiatrists concerned with psychotic patients, and changed institutions for the custodial care of mental patients into active treatment centers. Insulin therapy must also be credited with increasing efforts for the rehabilitation of psychiatric patients. It was possible for the first time to predict clinical changes, and social measures for the time after the patient's discharge could be undertaken with more promise of success.

Clinical research gained considerably. Psychological study of patients during the process of improvement contributed much to clinical knowledge. A methodology for statistical evaluation of results was established, based on various clinical and social yardsticks, whereby it was realized for the first time that evaluation procedures in psychiatry must use criteria different from those in other specialties of medicine. Prognostic studies became important, and prognostic tests prior to treatment were introduced. The interest in prognostication led to a less fatalistic attitude towards schizophrenia, for which hardly any prognostic studies had been available. Research in many different areas was stimulated by this new possibility to influence the course of a disease like schizophrenia, and this trend continued with the other treatment procedures that followed.

The use of insulin coma therapy spread widely and was soon considered the treatment of choice for schizophrenia. This continued to be so after the introduction of Metrazol and electric convulsive treatments. However, the use of insulin declined rapidly when the neuroleptic drugs were introduced. The reasons for this development were manifold. Some statistics showed unsatisfactory results, probably due to poor technique. Some dangers connected with its application were another reason for its unpopularity, although complications had become rare, when the termination of the hypoglycemic comas was simplified by means of the antiinsulinic pancreas hormone glucagon. Another reason might have been that the need for a lasting remission had become less pertinent since neuroleptic drugs permitted continued symptomatic treatment of the chronic schizophrenic. The main reason for the decline of insulin therapy was probably that it requires many months of labor by a great number of specially trained professionals. It is a strange paradox that, aside from the Soviet Union, some poor countries like India do not shy away from the greater efforts or higher expenses of insulin treatment and continue to use it. Many of us who have had experience with all biological treatments are convinced that insulin treatment, if given adequately, is the best treatment for schizophrenia, particularly if combined with the other methods that have become available since Sakel started his work.

By a strange coincidence, two other biological treatments were discovered almost at the same time. Only one year after Sakel's first publication in Vienna, the Hungarian psychiatrist, von Meduna, introduced another treatment for schizophrenia in neighboring Budapest and reported on his discovery in 1934. Again a clinical observation made in many mental hospitals was the point of origin for this new discovery. Mental patients who for one reason or another had spontaneous convulsions lost their symptoms quite dramatically, even though the symptoms returned later. The idea to use such convulsions therapeutically was further supported by some investigations suggesting that epilepsy and schizophrenia rarely occur in the same patient and, therefore, might eliminate each other. Prior to von Meduna, another Hungarian psychiatrist, Nyorö, had injected blood serum of epileptics into schizophrenic patients. When this had turned out to be ineffective, von Meduna took the next step and produced actual convulsive seizures in schizophrenics. Many means to induce seizures were available. Von Meduna chose camphor in oil; but this was rather slow and unreliable in producing a convulsive response, and he replaced it with intravenous injections of cardiazol, known in the United States as Metrazol. These Metrazol-induced convulsions led to dramatic changes in many patients. They did so much faster than insulin, although the convulsions had to be repeated many times in order to bring about a remission comparable to those obtained with insulin.

The overriding thought was the assumed antagonism between epilepsy and schizophrenia, and, therefore, metrazol convulsive therapy was recommended by Meduna exclusively for schizophrenia. However, a few years later it was particularly A. E. Bennett in this country who emphasized convulsive therapy for its great value in depressions. This illustrates the purely empirical discoveries in the history of biological treatments. Convulsive treatment continued to be useful in schizophrenia, although it turned out to be most effective in depressions, thus resembling the experience by Kuhn 20 years later, when he tried imipramine in schizophrenia and thereby discovered the most effective antidepressant drug.

Convulsive therapy today is mostly used in the form of electric convulsive therapy (ECT). It was quite accidental that Meduna chose pharmacological means to induce convulsions. A simpler and cleaner way to do this, even in experimental animals, had always been the electrical provocation of seizures. Therefore, it was not surprising that a few years later Cerletti and Bini introduced ECT. In the summer of 1937, Bini was the first to mention this work to the large International Treatment Conference organized in Münsingen, Switzerland, by Max Müller, who is still today an active force in biological treatments. In November 1937, the first patient was treated with ECT at the Psychiatric University Hospital in Rome, where I happened to work at that time. On March 15, 1938, Cerletti and Bini presented their method at the Academy of Medicine in Rome. The original fear of the electric current was noticeable from the fact that during this demonstration Bini failed several times to apply a sufficiently strong stimulus, which resulted in subconvulsive responsives before finally a grand mal seizure was obtained. The method soon spread to other countries, and two years later was accepted in the United States, in spite of a warning against possible electrocution in an editorial of the *Journal of the American Medical Association.*

The almost simultaneous appearance of two entirely different treatments for schizophrenia soon led to the combination of insulin coma and convulsive therapies. Such combinations became the most effective way to treat schizophrenia, although the first two pioneers, Sakel and Meduna, were inclined to limit themselves each to his own method. Later, both came to the United States, where Sakel continued to use insulin, while Meduna developed a new biological treatment, this time designed for the psychoneuroses. It consisted of carbon dioxide inhalation, applied to patients in repeated sessions and producing various degrees of unconsciousness. However, the results hardly went beyond what can be achieved in neurotic patients with many different means. The treatment was based on a biological theory of Meduna regarding the etiology of psychoneuroses. Carbon dioxide treatment never achieved in the neuroses anything comparable to the effect convulsive therapy has in the psychoses. Today it is almost given up, but Meduna will retain his place in the history of psychiatry as the originator of convulsive therapy.

Today, after 35 years, convulsive therapy is still widely used. ECT is a good example of how clinical experience alone decides on the actual value of treatment. Neither statistical comparison with other treatments, which often turned out to be contradictory, nor much-publicized side effects, nor objections by some psychiatrists on theoretical grounds and by the general public against something that is called "shock," stopped its use.

Efforts to avoid complications and side effects led to some fascinating research. In this country, A. E. Bennett embarked on brilliant investigations with curare, extracted from the South American plant *Chondodendron tomentosum* and used by Indian hunters to paralyze the muscles of animals. It appeared useful, therefore, for the prevention of ECT fractures due to muscular contractions. Later on, curare was abandoned because of its dangers, but the principle of the curare effect was upheld and is now obtained with the more innocuous succinyl choline, which entirely eliminates the possibility of fractures.

Another side effect of ECT, the unpleasant, although never-lasting memory impairment, opened up another avenue of research, which culminated in the use of unilaterally induced seizures. Historically, the first, though never-mentioned report to this effect was given by Thenon in Argentina in 1956. It was shown that unilateral stimulation of the nondominant hemisphere of the brain largely eliminates the patient's confusion that is so disturbing with the usual bilateral stimulation. Although the therapeutic effectiveness of this unilateral treatment is questioned, new ways toward an understanding of the effect of ECT have been opened up. Aside from such specific areas of research, convulsive therapy, like insulin, led to a host of other research investigations.

The eventful years between 1933 and 1938 brought still another treatment method into being. In Portugal, Moniz, in collaboration with Lima, performed the first surgical intervention on the frontal lobes of a schizophrenic patient by means of alcohol injections on November 12, 1935, and in December of the same year, destroyed the same fibers with a blunt instrument called a leukotome, thereby initiating the therapeutic approach later termed psychosurgery. Actually, brain operations in mental illness had already been reported in 1890 by the Swiss psychiatrist Burckhardt, and also by the Estonian psychosurgeon Puusepp around 1910. Both had discontinued their attempts, while Moniz proceeded with his work. It may be mentioned that he and Wagner-von Jauregg were the only neuropsychiatrists awarded the Nobel Prize.

The decisive figure in the propagation of psychosurgery, however, was an American, Walter Freeman, who, although not a surgeon, made, and is still making, the greatest contributions in this field. Prefrontal lobotomy was actually the most scientific discovery of any psychiatric treatment because it is based not only on clinical studies of frontal lobe lesions but also on intensive animal experimentation by men like Jacobsen and Fulton. They had noticed that bilateral interruption of connections of frontal lobe cortex and thalamus led to pronounced emotional changes reducing aggression. A similar effect was expected and found in the emotional response of psychiatric patients to their psychotic experiences after they had been operated on, and of neurotic patients to their anxieties and obsessive-compulsive preoccupations. The extensive use of this surgical approach in disturbed schizophrenics was mostly abandoned when the neuroleptic drugs were introduced. However, the complete rejection of psychosurgery was unjustified, and recently a definite upsurge is taking place in modified psychosurgical interventions for such psychiatric disorders as obsessive-compulsive neuroses, chronic depressions and other selected cases.

In concluding this historical survey, one should emphasize that the discovery of these biological treatments had an enormous impact on the whole field of psychiatry in both clinical work and research. We should realize that, contrary to all other fields of medicine, psychiatry deals mostly with diseases of which we do not know the cause but that we treat with increasing success by means of treatments that were found empirically and whose mechanisms we also do not understand. This is well illustrated by such divergent views on the etiology of psychiatric illness as prenatal factors, early childhood environment and, at the other end, pathophysiological and chemical changes in the brain. The appearance of effective treatments for these poorly understood diseases led to the hope that by finding the mode of action of these treatments in a manic-depressive or schizophrenic patient, we might in turn begin to understand their illness. So far, this expectation has remained unfulfilled for both the treatments I have discussed and also the new psychotropic drugs. However, research efforts in this direction continue, and I am convinced that finding common denominators in the various biological treatments will be the key to better understanding of the psychiatric disorders for which these treatments were devised.

CHAPTER

5

The Long Road For a Drug From Idea to Use

THE AMPHETAMINES

CHAUNCEY D. LEAKE, PHD*

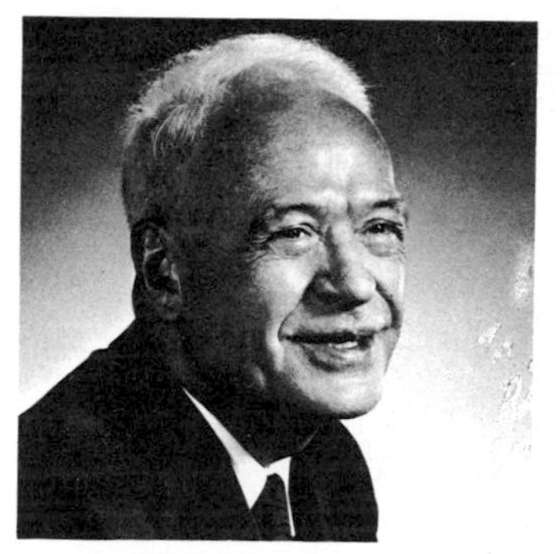

IT IS CHARACTERISTIC of the imaginative insight of Doctor Frank J. Ayd that he should have brought together so distinguished a group for the purpose of telling how a number of the currently used drugs of psychiatric interest were developed. It is important always to compile significant history as it occurs. Very striking indeed has been the development of extraordinary chemical agents for effects on our complicated brains and nervous systems. That many of them have become seriously abused is unfortunate, but with the vast numbers of our people, so many of whom have psychiatric problems, it is not to be wondered that wide and pathetic misuse of some of these agents should occur.

It would seem that it is most important to try to get as much information as we can to young people by groovy education on drug use, so that they will understand the dangers that there are in the abuse of these powerful new agents. Psychiatric drug abuse is a significant part of the current history of our overcrowded planet. Maybe we can learn to use these potent drugs more satisfactorily and effectively as we learn to reduce our numbers to fit more appropriately into our environment.

* Senior Lecturer, University of California, San Francisco 94122.

THE START IS OFTEN ACCIDENTAL

In World War I, I had left Princeton in 1917 to serve in a machinegun company. When the Chemical Warfare Service was organized, Doctor Harold C. Bradley (who later was one of my teachers and who is now my good friend in San Francisco) was personnel officer. When the Medical Defense Division was organized at the University of Wisconsin Medical School, I was assigned to this unit under Doctors Walter J. Meek (1878-1963) and Arthur S. Loevenhart (1878-1929). My job was to aid in the study of the physiological effects of various war gases on morphinized dogs, with particular references to changes in the blood acid-base equilibrium and other biochemical factors. When the war was over, I was asked to stay to study the effects of morphine. This would be the proper control.

This started my interest in the relief of pain. The problem of pain is a fascinating one, and of great importance psychiatrically. Some people are extremely sensitive to various stress factors that may produce either mental or physical pain, whereas other individuals are strangely resistant. I've come to the conclusion after pondering the various theories of "pain," that this is a word, a symbol, which simply means "too much." When the number of incoming stimuli from any part of the body reaches the point where the separate stimuli cannot be identified, the overall feeling is "pain." It is interesting that the afferent nervous system includes double feedback through an efferent nervous pathway in order to localize pain.

My studies led me to consider the mechanism of action of pain-relieving drugs. As to morphine, I concluded that it interferes with intracellular oxidation, probably in relation to various enzyme systems. Under these conditions, the brain cells involved would not function appropriately and probably impulses would not pass. In general, morphine is highly effective for the relief of traumatic pain, and if the dosage is large enough it will produce anesthesia. On the other hand, the various aromatic analgesics, such as aspirin, seem to act effectively in the relief of congestive pain, not only through a central pathway that may help lower temperature, but also peripherally by pulling fluid out of congested areas.

I felt that it would be interesting to try to develop a morphine compound that would relieve pain without addiction. This problem was later taken up by the US Public Health Service, and many millions of dollars were spent without significant result. My interest in the physiological effects of morphine, and my concern over the problem of pain, led me to undertake studies in anesthesia.

While at the University of Wisconsin, I worked on the effects of the common anesthetic agents on blood reaction. This was about the time when ethylene was introduced as an inhalation anesthetic by Arno Luckhardt (1885-1957) in Chicago. I found that ethylene does not produce as serious a disturbance in blood reaction as other inhalation anesthetic agents do, and this might correlate with its clinical advantages in producing less postoperative nausea and vomiting. Usually the general inhalation anesthetics, such as ether and chloroform, produce a ketotic diabetic condition. Nitrous oxide is effective only at high concentrations such as 90% at sea level, and this reduces the amount of oxygen that can be administered. With nitrous oxide there is a diphasic shift in blood reaction, with an initial alkalosis followed by an acidosis.

THE IDEAS BEGIN TO BE IMPLEMENTED

In 1928 I came to San Francisco to organize the pharmacology laboratory at the University of California, on the top floor of the old ivy-covered yellow-brick medical building on Parnassus Heights. We had a busy big room, and we soon had a group of keen youngsters on the job, led by Peter Knoefel (later Professor at the University of Louisville and now in Florence). With George Emerson, now Professor at the University of Texas in Galveston, we decided that we would try to reduce the respiratory depressant effects of morphine by combining the morphine molecule with an agent that would stimulate respiration. We used dinitrophenol, which had been developed by Doctor Maurice Tainter at Stanford Medical School in San Francisco, as an agent to stimulate oxidative metabolism. We made dinitrophenyl-morphine. This is pain relieving, and we had laboratory evidence to indicate that it might not be as addictive as morphine. However, we could not get the Federal bureaucrats to allow us to use it in humans and to determine whether or not it might be clinically valuable.

Later, with Elton McCawley (now Professor at the University of Oregon in Portland) and E. Leong Way (who is still at the University of California), we developed N-allyl-nor-morphine, or nalorphine. This we found to be a morphine antagonist. We hadn't developed it for that purpose, but that's what it turned out to be. It is now used to counteract morphine poisoning, and it is also employed widely to detect morphine or heroin addiction.

This was synthesized as a result of our studies showing that the allyl grouping has respiratory-stimulating effects. We were investigating various unsaturated ethers. As a result of my studies at the University of Wisconsin, I thought it might be a good idea to try to introduce the unsaturated carbon bonding of ethylene into the ether molecule. This would result in the compound divinyl ether. At the time it did not exist. Finally, I was able to obtain it from my friends at Princeton. Randolph Major, who later became research director for Merck and Company, prepared a considerable series of unsaturated symmetrical and unsymmetrical ethers. We found, as anticipated, that divinyl ether was the most satisfactory of the series. It was in this study that we found that the allyl compounds tend to have respiratory-stimulating effects. We found that divinyl ether is a useful inhalation anesthetic agent. It is rapid and powerful. It is used especially in children, and for induction. I was surprised to learn last year that it is especially popular in Scandanavia. It is gratifying, but also most puzzling, to realize that one may devise a chemical compound to relieve the certain pain of surgery without knowing what pain is or how the chemical agent acts!

On the other hand, we also learned that on prolonged administration divinyl ether may injure the liver. Furthermore it is flammable. We tried to halogenate the compound in order to reduce flammability. We could obtain many different chlorinated and brominated saturated and unsaturated ethers, but none was satisfactory. We thought, of course, about fluorine, but at the time no chemists were able satisfactorily to handle fluorine.

This problem of the halogenated saturated and unsaturated ethers for anesthesia was studied vigorously by my good friend, John Krantz, of the University of Maryland in Baltimore. He was able to obtain fluorinated compounds. He found several that were promising and useful, and one that was remarkable in that it might produce central nervous stimulation instead of depression. This study culminated in the success of Imperial Chemical Industries in England under James Bogue, in obtaining tri-fluro-brom-chlor-ethane. This is the now popular "halothane (Fluothane)," a rapid and highly effective inhalation anesthetic agent and not flammable or explosive.

An interesting side-development of our studies on anesthesia came while I was still at the University of Wisconsin, working with Ralph M. Waters, who developed the first important anesthesia training center in the United States, laying the foundation for the now great specialty of anesthesiology. He was interested in removing carbon dioxide from patients during prolonged anesthesia. This was successfully solved by using soda lime. Since the general inhalation anesthetic agents are metabolized very slightly in the body once a patient is satisfactorily anesthetized, it is only necessary to maintain that concentration of the anesthetic agent, and then supply oxygen as the patient requires it, removing the carbon dioxide that has formed. Waters and Art Guedel successfully applied clinically, the experimental demonstration made by Dennis Jackson of Cincinnati.

We became interested in carbon dioxide, since a century before, in 1828, Henry Hill Hickman (1800-1830) in England found that carbon dioxide causes anesthesia in dogs. He thought it might be used clinically, but his idea was met with scorn, and he killed himself in despair. A century later, Ralph Waters and I took up the matter and found that carbon dioxide is a satisfactory general inhalation anesthetic agent in dogs, administered in a concentration of 30% carbon dioxide with 70% oxygen. Under these circumstances there is no possibility of anoxic effects. The maintainence of anesthesia, however, is likely to be a little stormy, so that carbon dioxide anesthesia was never seriously considered clinically.

On the other hand, we had noted that in recovery from carbon dioxide anesthesia, in our experimental animals, there is some evidence of delirium. This frequently occurs with other anesthetic agents. It is interesting that there had already been clinical observations that during recovery from inhalation anesthesia, schizophrenic patients may show a short lucid interval.

I had the idea that we might employ carbon dioxide in a concentration of 30% with 70% oxygen in schizophrenic patients. Accordingly, when I came to San Francisco, I arranged with Mary Botsford, the anesthetist at the University of California, and Arthur E. Guedel, the distinguished anesthetist from Los Angeles, to make the trial on schizophrenic patients.

We went to the Agnew State Hospital for our study. I well remember our first patient. He was a huge strapping black man in a catatonic state. He gave negative responses by clenching his fists and shutting his eyes tightly on questioning, so that we knew he was responsive. Upon the administration of 30% carbon dioxide and

70% oxygen, he took several deep breaths, sat up, opened his eyes, looked around, and asked where he was. He smiled when we said that we were trying to help him, and then almost immediately his eyes began to glaze over, and within a minute he was back in his former catatonic state.

We went on with seven more schizophrenic patients. In each we were able to produce a short period of mental clarity, so that questions were answered intelligently, and so that the individuals seemed to be alert and responsive to their environment in what seemed to be a normal way. In no case, however, was the effect prolonged. Later, Ladislas Meduna of Chicago continued to study carbon dioxide administration in schizophrenic patients, and went from this to the use of convulsive therapy employing metrazol. He was no more successful than we were, even on long-continued and frequent administrations of carbon dioxide, to induce any prolonged improvement in schizophrenic patients.

My interest in pain and anesthesia has continued. There are still many ideas that may helpfully be developed from the information we now have regarding the relation between chemical constitution and biological action. This field, which we labeled "biochemorphology," was a major concern in our laboratory at the University of California, and now it is attracting much wider interest than forty years ago.

PSYCHIATRIC ASPECTS OF INTESTINAL DISORDERS

Shortly after we established the pharmacology group at the University of California, San Francisco, we were asked by our colleagues in the Hooper Foundation for Medical Research, under the direction of Professor K. F. Meyer, to undertake a chemotherapeutic survey of amebiasis. This remains a widespread disease, with a high incidence in the tropics, but tending to fade away towards the more temperate areas. Nevertheless, a survey in our own San Francisco area showed that about 10% of the population carried amebic cysts. The drugs commonly in use, one an organic arsenical and the other a hydroxyquinoline, were not particularly satisfactory.

We were able to make a survey of many organic arsenical derivatives, with a grant of $3,000 a year for about five years from Eli Lilly. We had a similar grant from Ciba for a survey of the halogenated hydroxyquinolines. We were able to establish a broad method for estimating toxicity both on single and repeated administration, for examination of the organs of the body to determine what might be injured, and then to survey not only the general pharmacological actions of the compounds in which we were interested, but also their specific chemotherapeutic effect in natural amebiasis in macaques. We carefully studied the rates of absorption and excretion of these compounds.

We were fortunate in finding a couple that have survived in clinical usefulness to this day. One is carbarsone, an organic arsenical compound, widely used in treating active amebiasis. The other is Vioform, or 5-chloro-7-iodo-8-hydroxyquinoline. This agent is not absorbed from the intact intestinal tract and has practically no toxicity; it is highly effective in relatively small dosage of about 500 mgm per day for 10 days.

Vioform was widely introduced for use around the world. Travelers presently found that it was helpful in relieving the distressing symptoms of unexplained diarrheas that cause so much distress among people in the warmer lands. Later studies showed that it is highly effective in clearing the intestinal tract of a number of bacterial as well as protozoal invaders. It has been found particularly effective in shigella infections. It is available for over-the-counter purchase in all countries of the world except the United States. Why it is that our Food and Drug Administration continues to require people to get a doctor's prescription and go through all the red tape and expense necessary to obtain the drug is a mystery to me. It is effective, and it is safe. What more does the Food and Drug Administration want?

The distress of diarrheas when traveling can produce severe psychological disturbance. With continued fixation on the intestinal tract, people can become psychotic. We feel that we have been able to relieve the minds of many travelers, and indeed of many people who live in the tropics by making available worthwhile drugs for their use. While it is true that many natives in tropical areas seem to be immune from the ordinary diarrheas that distress travelers, many natives nevertheless do suffer from chronic and mild diarrheal conditions. This may be associated with malnutrition; indeed, malnutrition and diarrheas go together, and often which is cause and which effect is not apparent.

Native peoples all over the world have learned to use barks and other materials that contain tannins for the relief of diarrheas.

Many of these have been assumed to be specific for amebiasis. This is not the case. Any agent that contains tannin or gums or resins in sufficient quantity may help to coat over the insides of the intestinal tract and thus allay irritation and reduce the diarrheal condition. The ease of mind that may come from the use of an effective antidiarrheal agent is, I think, an important contribution to the prevention of psychoses.

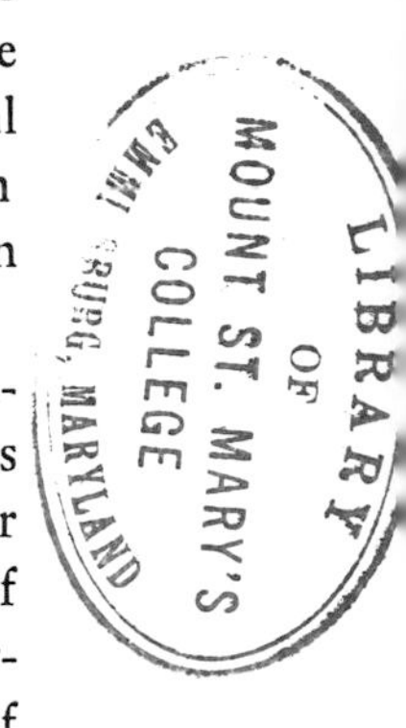

Much of the work on carbarsone was carried through by Hamilton Anderson, who later studied its effectiveness on field expeditions in various parts of the world. He is now a toxicology consultant for government agencies in Hawaii as well as for the University of Hawaii. Many of the studies on vioform were conducted by Norman David, now professor of Pharmacology at the University of Oregon in Portland. He also aided greatly in the field studies on vioform, which established its clinical effectiveness.

THE AMPHETAMINES

Among the many impecunious but hardworking young people who came to our laboratory was Myron Prinzmetal, from Los Angeles. He worked on mussel and shell-fish poison, and began studies on respiratory and cardiac conditions that he continued so effectively later. One day he told me that he had a good friend in Los Angeles, Gordon Alles (1901-1963), who was a chemist in the clinical office of George Piness. There he was making a series of purified proteins for use in testing for allergy.

Ephedrine had been introduced as an effective agent against asthma when given by mouth. This was based on the brilliant studies of my long-time friend, Dr. K. K. Chen, who had been with me at the University of Wisconsin and was a pupil of Dr. Harold Bradley. Later he obtained his medical degree from the Johns Hopkins University. Returning to China, he began a systematic investigation of the ancient Chinese drug codification, and noticed the repeated reoccurrence of a desert plant, Ma Huang, as a treatment for asthma. Looking into the matter, he discovered that it was the plant, *Ephedra vulgaris*, from which the alkaloid ephedrine can be obtained. Ephedrine is closely related chemically to epinephrine, the chemical agent formed in the adrenal medulla, which, in the emergency theory of Walter Cannon (1871-1947), prepares an animal for "fight or flight," by raising blood pressure, dilating the bronchi, relaxing the gut, and dilating the pupils. Ephedrine was widely used in the treatment of asthma, and the native supplies were exhausted. George Piness suggested to Gordon Alles, his chemist, that an attempt be made to find a synthetic substitute for ephedrine.

Gordon Alles prepared a number of related phenyl-alkyl-amine compounds and was seeking an opportunity to study their biological activity. He had no satisfactory place available in southern California. Under these circumstances, Myron Prinzmetal suggested that I invite Gordon Alles to come and work in our laboratory. Gordon Alles came and regularly spent about a month every quarter of the year in our laboratory, systematically studying the biological activity of the different compounds he had made. He was meticulous in his effort. In all cases, he prepared solutions with extreme care, and used them on an equimolecular basis, so that he could properly compare one agent with another. The toxicity studies were made on single and repeated administration, usually on small animals, in order to obtain statistically valid results. The general biological actions were studied carefully on larger animals.

The most effective agent that Alles was able to find in his series of compounds was phenyl-isopropyl-amine. This he called "benzedrine." At first he used the racemic compound. Making this into the carbonate, he found that it was volatile and thus could be inhaled. This afforded a means for the rapid relief of an acute asthmatic attack. The drug was widely developed by Smith Kline & French laboratories in Philadelphia and it was given the public name "amphetamine." In the studies on levo and dextro isomers of amphetamine, Gordon Alles found that dextro compound, "dexedrine," is a powerful central nervous system (CNS) stimulant. The general CNS-stimulating effect of amphetamine had been noted early.

In studying the compound on himself, Gordon Alles found that amphetamine would tend to prolong wakefulness, increase alertness, and generally stimulate the CNS. The drug was introduced clinically by Myron Prinzmetal, and also by Anderson Peoples, who also worked in our laboratory and had gone to London for clinical work in psychiatry at the Maudsley Hospital. There he successfully used amphetamine in the treatment of narcolepsy, and it became widely employed for this purpose. It was soon found that amphetamine also would tend to reduce appetite, and as a result it began to be used clinically for the treatment of obesity.

Amphetamine is effective by mouth and is one of the most useful

CNS stimulants. It tends to relieve fatigue, and it became very widely used in combating sleepiness and depression. During World War II, amphetamine was used by the German Panzer troops. A modification of amphetamine was also employed. This was the methyl-amine derivative known generally as meth-amphetamine. When I suggested that our troops be supplied with amphetamine to combat fatigue and to maintain alertness, I was overruled on the claim by A. C. Ivy that amphetamine might be too toxic for this purpose. Actually the British aviators used it in order to keep awake in their long bombing missions. Our aviators bootlegged it from the British. The Japanese used methamphetamine extensively also among their troops.

At the end of World War II, Japan had large stocks of meth-amphetamine, which were dumped on the open market. In Japan most all drugs are available over-the-counter in drug stores, excepting morphine, cocaine and heroin. The Japanese are very sophisticated about drugs and health affairs, and their drugs are very well packaged with full information as to what the drugs will do and what their dangers are. Furthermore, pharmacists usually aid in self-medication. When World War II was over, many of the Japanese youngsters found it very difficult to get along with the meager salaries they were able to earn during the day. The result is that most of them moonlighted with jobs at night. In order to keep awake, they took meth-amphetamine. A very widespread use of the drug under these conditions uncovered a considerable number of latent psychoses. This was the first indication that the amphetamines might be subject to abuse.

It was shocking to learn in connection with the drug culture in the Haight-Ashbury district of San Francisco, that meth-amphetamine was beginning to be obtained on the blackmarket and used by vein. This is certainly something we never anticipated. It was badly abused. The abuse of amphetamine was widely extended by blackmarket racketeering. The extent of this was revealed by Margaret Kreig in her book, *Blackmarket Medicine*, which appeared in 1967. The pattern of amphetamine abuse followed that of many other addictive drugs. It remains a question in my mind whether or not the amphetamines are truly addictive in the sense of producing the same kind of physical dependence characteristic of morphine.

Much of the abuse of the amphetamines involves the widespread use of depressant drugs, particularly the sleep-producing barbitals. The use of the barbitals has increased extensively throughout our country in response to the increased tension of modern living. Unfortunately, people tend to go on the principle that if a little bit of a drug is good for what you wish it to do, a little bit more is better, which is always dangerous. The barbitals tend to have a much more lasting effect than ordinarily thought. Consequently, with work to be done in the morning, and with a hangover of depression from the sleeping agent that was taken the night before, many people began to use amphetamines to stimulate them and keep them awake, a bad whipsaw situation. Unfortunately, many people fell into this trap.

The abuse of the amphetamines seriously distressed Gordon Alles and all of us who had been concerned in their development. It was apparent that high doses of the amphetamines could produce a CNS disturbance to the point of minor hallucination. It seems that some of the "kick" desired by those who inject amphetamine results from this partial hallucinating effect. Alles studied many derivatives of the amphetamines in our laboratory. These he had made in his own laboratory, which he was able to establish in Los Angeles. One of these derivatives, a methylene-dioxy-phenyl-alkyl-amine was found to have an extraordinary effect in producing a time differential in perception between a sensory stimulus such as a touch on the skin and the sight of that touch. After taking this drug, if one would hit one's finger, one could see the strike at the finger, but feel it later. It was found that this was not due to a slowing of nerve-conduction from the finger through the spinal cord to the brain, but rather a disturbance in the correlation between sight and touch occurring in the brain itself.

We had much interest in our laboratory in connection with hallucination. We had hoped to be able to develop a systematic study of hallucinating drugs in general. Meanwhile, however, the Haight-Ashbury scene had taken over and the whole matter of hallucinating agents was in the open. We felt that Gordon Alles' studies on the amphetamines had opened for us a wide new vista into the action of drugs on the central nervous system.

THE DRUG THAT DID NOT DELIVER

There is currently a great deal of discussion about various moral aspects of human experimentation. This is complicated by much of the technical requirements in respect to drugs for control of bias or subjective opinion, and has resulted in the general development of the double- or triple-blind study. The problem still remains, however, about telling the truth to the human subjects who may be required for effective testing of a new drug before it goes into general clinical use. There are legal as well as moral problems involved. Often it is thought that, if the human subjects for drug experimentation sign a consent form, all is clear. This has no legal standing. If an individual who has been used for experimental studies of a new drug should feel that he or she might have been injured, there is nothing to prevent his bringing a suit for damage. On the other hand, the consent form may actually make the clinical pharmacologist or clinical experimenter feel that all is safe and that it is not necessary to use the exceptional extreme care and caution in carrying forward this study that might be required if there were liability for injury.

There is often a conflict of ethical theory in the situation. It is astonishing how we all assume that we all follow the same general ethical principles. Actually there are some two dozen theories of ethics and most of us find it convenient to change from one to the other as we rationalize our conduct. In the case of the clinical trials for new drugs, the subject is usually motivated by a desire to help do something for humanity in general: to serve as a willing sacrifice as it were for the benefit of society. This is social idealism. On the other hand, the experimenter is usually a pragmatist and is interested simply in whether or not the experiment works out. If it does, it's all to the good. If money is involved, as it usually is, there is a hedonistic element in that all parties concerned are eager to get as much money out of the situation as possible, even though they may disguise their motives in many ways.

Further, it is always to be remembered that any procedure that is conducted by a member of the health professions or services is an experiment. It doesn't matter whether the procedure is diagnostic, preventative, curative, or merely the alleviation of symptoms. The outcome cannot be predicted with certainty. While most of us fall on the high portion of the Gaussian or bell-shaped distribution curve, it is always the few at the extreme ends that make the trouble. Using the same drug at the same dosage, some people may show no effect at all, while others may give results that are extremely dangerous or may even result in death.

This is to be expected if enough individuals are studied. Thus it is in the mass use of vaccines with large numbers of people. When oral polio vaccine was introduced into Canada, it was used first on some two million youngsters. Four died. The situation was such that the deaths could have been ascribed to the vaccine. Nevertheless, the authorities went ahead with general mass vaccination on the basis of the greatest good for the greatest number. Most of us would be willing to take one chance in 500,000. The social benefit to be derived from the mass vaccination with polio would be more important than the possible injury to a relatively few individuals. So it is with almost all chemicals.

In our own laboratory, we made it a point always to use our new drugs on ourselves first, if we thought that the experimental evidence was sufficient to indicate that they might have value. We felt reasonably secure. We had covered all aspects of toxicity that we could think of on single and repeated administration, including pathological examination of animals that might be sacrificed. Further we had as clear evidence as could be obtained about the effects of the drug on various parts of the body and on the overall picture. This worked well with the drugs I have so far described. However, there was one drug that did not work out.

We became interested in furan derivatives. The furan organic radical is even more aromatic than benzene. We thought that we could make the furan analogs of all the major benzene compounds then in common use. We first made some furan antiseptics. They worked out well, and they are still in general use. We then tried furan local anesthetics, and we could make them readily also. However, there is no interest in new local anesthetics. They remain a dime a dozen, and there's no particular point in trying to develop one on account of the lack of commercial interest.

I then thought it might be worthwhile to see if we could develop a furan aspirin. Aspirin is, after the alcoholic beverages, the most widely used drug all over the world. Its toxicity is well established; its usefulness is also well established. It is an excellent agent for the relief of congestive pain. We made a furan aspirin. It had satisfactory physical-chemical properties; it is absorbed readily by mouth, and it seems to be metabolized quickly, at about the same rate as aspirin itself. We found, on experimental study, that it will lower the temperature in a variety of experimental fevers, and we also had good evidence that it will reduce congestive swelling.

Under these circumstances, it might have been expected to be a useful drug for the relief of congestive pain. Our toxicity studies, in a variety of animals, showed that it was nontoxic on single administration and even on repeated administration of large doses. However, we did not look carefully enough.

When I thought that we had satisfactory evidence for the usefulness of the furan aspirin, I conveniently had a headache and thought I'd better try it on myself. I did so in the usual aspirin dosage. My headache seemed to go away and I felt quite elated. The next day I thought again that I had a headache and took double the dosage that I had before. Again the headache went away and I thought that now we were in business. I thought we'd probably be able to subsidize the laboratory from then on. But in order to make sure, on the next morning, I took another dose of the furan aspirin. Then I noticed something. I had difficulty in urinating: it was extremely painful; I wound up in the hospital and found that the drug had precipitated in the inside of my bladder and while not irritating there, it nevertheless seriously interfered with urination. We had failed to observe this kind of effect in our animals. They can't talk.

Nevertheless, furan aspirin never got beyond me. Nobody else in fact has ever taken it. It seems to me that this is the way in which to handle the matter of clinical trial. If you're really interested in a drug, use it on yourself first.

LOOKING AHEAD

I have described several drugs that are of interest in psychiatric conditions from idea to delivery, pointing out that in one instance, there was no delivery for the good and sufficient reason that the drug did not work out on human trial. Those were pleasant days. We could carry through our work using our own standards and our own criteria. After all, there were not too many of us to get in each other's way. Now that there are so many of us, we have such a variety of regulatory agencies, local, state, and federal, that it is extremely difficult to try to develop any new chemical compound to the point of effective delivery. It takes a vast organization; it requires a tremendous amount of money; it is hedged in with an enormous amount of red tape; the results are not impressive.

There are minor psychiatric overtones to all of this. Those who become involved, either from the standpoint of the development of new drugs or from the standpoint of regulating this development, tend to become neurotic. Those who are interested in developing the new drugs tend to feel that they are being harassed and interfered with by the authoritarians who operate within the regulations. Those who are in authority tend to display it. The result is unfortunate.

Unfortunate also is the fact that our laws tend towards absolutes. Current laws regulating the development of new drugs seem to imply absolute safety and absolute effectiveness. There is no chemical at all that will meet these two conditions, not even table salt or common water. We badly need to get ourselves together in understanding that cooperative endeavor for the benefit of all would inevitably help each. We should always remember also that responsible individual endeavor that may result in individual advancement usually, if it is responsible, will be of benefit to all. Under these circumstances, it might be possible for us to work out a little more satisfactory leeway in connection with the development of new drugs from ideas to delivery.

I'm an old man and I've seen many changes in connection with the development of new drugs. This has ranged from the time when the toxicity of a drug might be estimated on the basis of 3 out of 5 deaths in small animals for what was then called the "minimum lethal dosage," to highly sophisticated techniques of estimating dosage and of assuring the toxic range in a wide variety of animals, always controlled with full pathological postmortem examination. But we can't think of everything.

I gave an illustration in my own experience in connection with the furan aspirin. The thalidomide fiasco was of a similar sort. We've had trouble before. When ethylene glycol was introduced as an effective organic solvent, it was used as a vehicle for sulfanilamide, without testing the toxicity of the solvent. After there were many deaths, it was realized that ethylene glycol is itself seriously toxic.

Meanwhile, I have seen all sorts of sophisticated efforts made to work out satisfactory information on new drugs from idea to delivery. This will continue. We're never satisfied with what we have. This may be slightly psychiatric in itself. However, as long as we are committed to the shibboleth of progress, we probably will continue to try always to get something better than we have. Maybe this, after all, is best for us all.

There is enormous interest in chemical agents that can alter the exquisitely balanced chemical equilibrium of our brains. We continue to learn from such drugs how our brains may work, in health and disease. But our ignorance remains appalling. Even after millenia of experience with alcoholic beverages, we don't know how they produce their effects, pleasurable if used in moderation, disastrous when used in excess. Our effective use of stimulating and depressing drugs remains empirical. Yet, by following biochemorphic, or structure-action relationships, we can continue to develop safer and more satisfactory drugs for psychiatric use.

REFERENCES

Carbon-dioxide anesthesia, and effectiveness in schizophrenia:

1. Leake, C. D., and Waters, R. M.: J Pharmacol Exp Ther *33:*280, 1928; Anesth Analg (Cleveland) *8:*17-19, 1929;
2. Leake, C. D., Guedel, A. E., and Botsford, M. E.: Calif Med *31:*20-24, 1929.

Divinyl ether:

1. Leake, C. D., and Chen, Mei-yu: Proc Soc Exp Biol Med *28:*151-154, 1930;
2. Leake, C. D., Knoefel, P. K., and Guedel, A. E.: J Pharmacol Exp Ther *47:*5-16, 1933;
3. Leake, C. D.: JAMA *102:*1-4, (Jan 6), 1934.

Chemotherapy of amebiasis:

1. Leake, C. D.: JAMA *98:*195-198 (Jan 16), 1932;
2. Reed, A. C., Anderson, H. H., David, N. A., and Leake, C. D.: JAMA *98:*189-194 (Jan 16), 1932;
3. David, N. A., Johnstone, H. G., Reed, A. C., Leake, C. D.: JAMA *100:* 1658-1661 (May 27), 1933.

The amphetamines:

1. Alles, G. A.: J Pharmacol Exp Ther *47:*339-354, 1933;
2. Alles, G. A., and Prinzmetal, M.: J Pharmacol Exp Ther *48:*161-174, 1933;
3. Peoples, S. A., and Guttmann, E.: Lancet *1:*1107-1109 (May 16), 1936;
4. Prinzmetal, M., and Bloomberg, W.: JAMA *105:*2051-2055, 1935;
5. Alles, G. A., and Knoefel, P. K.: Univ Calif Pub, Pharmacol *1:*101-118, 1938;
6. Abreu, B. E., and Handley, C. A.: Univ Calif Pub, Pharmacol *2:*99-104, 1942;
7. Alles, G. A., and Feigen, G. A.: Amer J Physiol *136:*392-400, 1942;
8. Leake, C. D.: The Amphetamines: Their Actions and Uses, Springfield (Ill), Thomas, 1958;
9. Alles, G. A.: Trans 4th Conf on Neuropharmacology, Macy Foundation, New York, 1959, pp. 181-268.

Dinitrophenyl morphine and N-allyl-normorphine:

1. Emerson, G. A., Klyza, S. J., Phatak, N. M., and Leake, C. D.: Univ Calif Pub, Pharmacol *1:*59-68, 69-76, 1938;

2. Abreu, B. E., Phatak, N. M., Emerson, G. A., and Leake, C. D.: Univ Calif Pub, Pharmacol *1*:77-92, 1938;
3. McCawley, E. L., and Hart, R. E.: J Amer Chem Soc *63*:314-316, 1941; J Phamacol Exp Ther 82:339-348, 1944;
4. Way, E. L.: Ass Res Neurol Ment Dis *46*:13-31, 1967.

Furan derivatives:

1. Phatak, N. M., and Leake, C. D.: J Pharmacol Exp Ther *56*:265-268, 1936; *58*:155-158, 1936.

CHAPTER

6

The Demonstration of the Specific Anticonvulsant Action of Diphenylhydantoin and Related Compounds

TRACY J. PUTNAM, MD, FAPA *

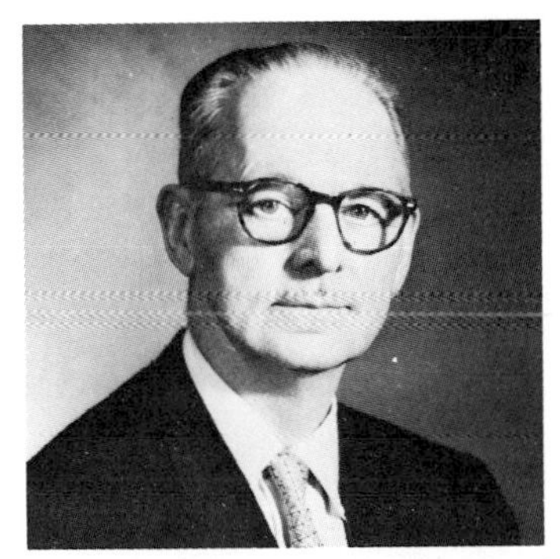

WHEN I WAS A STUDENT IN MEDICAL school a half century or more ago, the subject of epilepsy was given scant and poorly organized attention. In the course on Pediatrics, we were shown a few children having seizures but told nothing about neurophysiology or treatment. In the course on Neurology, we had a brief lecture on the clinical aspects of epilepsy. Osler's *Textbook* was our bible and this amazing work devoted a few pages to the subject, lifted almost verbatim from Hippocrates.

As it happened, I had more than a casual interest in the subject. When I was a boy, I learned that a relative of mine, whom I saw occasionally, suffered from epilepsy. I remember well the bromide pustules about his nose, and I remember being told that he had become an alcoholic because of his affliction. Although he was charming, intelligent, well educated and wealthy, he had become a lonely recluse. Shortly before I entered medical school, I witnessed the opening act of another tragedy due to epilepsy. This time the

* Beverly Hills, California.

victim was a close cousin, whom I regarded almost as a sister. She also became shut off from the world; half her colon was removed in an effort to relieve her attacks; finally she was somewhat better when given a new drug called Luminal. She underwent psychiatric treatment and this also appeared to improve her condition.

Looking further in the literature available to me, I learned that convulsions were sometimes apparently the result of wounds or tumors of the brain. In many cases, however, no physical cause could be found, and the most modern belief of that time was that the seizures were the result of a fundamental character defect, constituting a substitute for an excessive temper tantrum.

In 1923, I began a more intensive training in neurology, as a resident under Dr. Harvey Cushing. Devoted as he was to all patients suffering from brain tumors, he dreaded contact with epileptics who showed no neurological deficits. If one such were by accident admitted to his service, the patient was put at once on Luminal and discharged. I use the word Luminal with intent; during this residency, I prescribed phenobarbital for a patient, and the nurse on the case administered the prescribed dose of barbital, never having heard of the new-fangled nostrum. The patient awoke a few days later, and no lasting damage was done.

In the late 20's, I began to realize that the cases of epilepsy not susceptible to surgical treatment enormously outnumbered the ones with no localizing signature. At that time, the most dependable treatise on the subject was that by Lennox and Cobb, two good friends of mine. The only treatment recommended was the use of phenobarbital, and this without much enthusiasm. In the early 1930s, Dr. Lennox published his observation that in susceptible patients, seizures could often be produced by intentional hyperventilation producing acapnia. He showed also that attacks of petit mal might be inhibited by rebreathing in and out of a bag, or the administration of carbon dioxide.

About this time also, attention was being paid to the use of the ketogenic diet and starvation in the treatment of epilepsy. Dr. Lennox fasted for two weeks before suggesting this treatment to a patient. His first subject was a girl in her 20s who had suffered from frequent petit mal attacks for many years. After a two week fast, she became and remained seizure-free. The follow-up on this case could scarcely be surpassed, for the patient was an employee in the laboratory. Further, the idea of operative treatment of structural defects of the brain associated with seizures was revived. Such operations have been carried out for roughly a century, and it is striking to the inquiring observer that the more promptly the results are reported, the better they are. Often the patient was put on phenobarbital for the first time after the craniotomy. Osler's *Textbook* records that some 30 different types of operation, not necessarily on the head, have been reported to alleviate seizures.

In 1934, it became clear to me that I should do well to consider the possibility that the medical treatment of various neurological diseases might be improved. Important among these was clearly epilepsy. From consideration of the information just outlined, I felt that there was a biochemical component in the total etiology of convulsions and similar phenomena. A possible clue to a conceivable treatment was Dr. Lennox' observation that inhalation of carbon dioxide inhibited seizures. Might an institution for the treatment of epilepsy be established adjacent to a brewery, and the content of carbon dioxide in the atmosphere metered so as to be tolerable and yet sufficient to prevent attacks? The more I thought about this project, the worse it seemed.

Another possibility might be to isolate the "ketone bodies" presumably generated by the ketogenic diet and fasting and to administer them as such to the patient. At that time, I could not visualize the necessary steps, but perhaps something of the sort might now be feasible. As I pondered various approaches to the problem, it seemed to me that the most practical avenue might be to find an analogue of phenobarbital that, hopefully, could be less hypnotic and more powerful as an anticonvulsant. Obviously, from my own observation and data in the literature, phenobarbital was more effective than any other commonly used barbiturate, and presumably this is because it contains a phenol radical. While the whole project was in the speculative stage, I had an opportunity to discuss it with my old friend, Dr. Tinsley Harrison. He pointed out to me that convulsions are frequently seen in uremic states, but they do not occur if there is a high concentration of conjugated phenols in the bloodstream. The ideal for which to strive seemed then, to be a chemical substance containing one or more phenyl radicals attached to a ring or possibly an aliphatic group, more or less analogous to phenobarbital and to endogenous phenyl compounds. But if such a compound were found, how could it be tested?

The project was brought a step further when I assumed directorship of the Neurological Unit of the Boston City Hospital in 1934. Here I had laboratory space and animal quarters. More important, I had the help of Dr. Frederic Gibbs, who was engaged in setting up the first electroencephalographic laboratory in the world for routine clinical use. In this laboratory it became perfectly clear that every true seizure is attended by an electrical "storm" in the brain. It seemed likely, therefore, that a convulsion might be produced by applying a current to the brain, and possible that a convulsive threshold might be established by quantitating the current required. (I did not know it at that time, but later learned that Dr. Ernest Spiegel had devised a sophisticated apparatus for this purpose.) Accordingly Dr. Gibbs, Dr. Paul Hoefer and I assembled a rather crude quantitative stimulator that would measure the convulsive threshold in animals. Dr. Hoefer contributed not only advice, but a commutator salvaged from a World War I German airplane. Cats were chosen for experimental animals. A first trial showed that a well-tolerated dose of phenobarbital would raise the convulsive threshold about four times. I acquired also the invaluable technical assistance of Mrs. Dorothy Schwab, who had helped me over the years in most of my scientific studies: I doubt whether I could have brought them to fruition without her.

Next, I combed the Eastman Chemical Company's catalog, and other price lists, for suitable phenyl compounds that were not obviously poisonous. I also wrote to the major pharmaceutical firms, asking if they had available or could make suitable chemicals. The only one of them that showed any interest was Parke Davis and Company. They wrote back to me that they had on hand samples of 19 different compounds analogous to phenobarbital and that I was welcome to them. They added that this was probably a waste of time, for the compounds had been thoroughly tested and were inactive. Among the 19 was diphenylhydantoin. The others were indeed inactive. This one was clearly superior to phenobarbital, nonhypnotic and, apparently nontoxic. Meanwhile, a hundred-odd other substances had been tested, and a few of them appeared to have some anticonvulsant properties. All except diphenylhydantoin had disagreeable side effects and were discarded.

I did not seek patent protection for my observations, and they are in the public domain. Each time since then when I have approached bankruptcy, I have deeply regretted this noble renunciation; also each time I have seen a promising scientific project abandoned for lack of a few thousand dollars. I shall never cease to remember my personal indebtedness to Mr. Jack Dreyfus, whose generosity rescued me from the imminent prospect of a financially distressed old age. My wife and I have plans to amplify his gift, combine it with whatever other funds we may be able to accumulate, and eventually to leave it to further the scientific aims that have seemed so important to both of us.

To return to my story, about 1936 it became clear to me that the project was too large for the existing team, for many other things were going on at the Neurological Unit then. The Department of Electroencephalography was growing by leaps and bounds; Dr. Hoefer and I introduced electromyography into routine neurological practice for the first time. Dr. Donald Munro popularized the use of tidal drainage of the urinary bladder in neurological diseases. We were achieving some success with the surgical treatment of hydrocephalus, paralysis agitans, and athetosis. My studies on the pathogenesis of multiple sclerosis, begun in 1928, were at last taking definite form. The therapeutic uses of benzedrine were being explored. All of this seemed important and urgent at the time, although now, some thirty-odd years later, it seems clear to me that our endeavors have been completely forgotten or at all events ignored.

To return to 1936—I therefore asked Dr. H. Houston Merritt to join us. He was then my faithful Chef de Clinique, in charge of the Out-Patient Department, and as soon as reasonable toxicity experiments had been carried out, it seemed natural to request him to supervise the administration of diphenylhydantoin. He accordingly did so. Our first patient was a man who had been completely incapacitated for years because he suffered one or more seizures daily, unrelieved by phenobarbital. He has remained seizure-free since.

It was the policy of my department at Harvard to push young men forward. When time for publication came, I suggested to Dr. Merritt that I should be the senior author in publishing the experimental results in the *Archives of Neurology* but that his name should come first on the article on our clinical results. As events turned out, the latter was read by him at the American Medical Association meeting in San Francisco in 1938, and published in the *JAMA*. Dr. Merritt's subsequent career and succession to one of my chairs at Columbia University is a matter of history. He also became Dean of the College of Physicians and Surgeons at Columbia. The Dreyfus Award was presented to me, however, in 1969, through Harvard.

The announcement of our results was followed by bitter attacks from many sides. In the long run, it was apparently the insistent demand of uncounted patients that forced the medical profession to adopt the new idea. Years afterwards, textbooks of pharmacology were still stating that epilepsy should be treated with sedatives, and that phenobarbital had no advantages over other barbiturates.

Diphenylhydantoin has been found to have many actions and uses besides that for which it was originally selected. It has come into further use in psychiatry and cardiology, for example, and has been found experimentally to hasten the healing of wounds. Possibly even more uses for it may be found in the future.

A final comment: Had the present regulations of the Federal Drug Administration been in effect when this project was initiated, I doubt whether diphenylhydantoin would ever have reached the market. I know of still another drug, apparently effective in the control of seizures, which is lying unused and may well be lost because so far, no one has been willing to undertake the necessary financing.

CHAPTER

7

The Discovery of LSD and Subsequent Investigations on Naturally Occurring Hallucinogens

ALBERT HOFMANN, PHD *

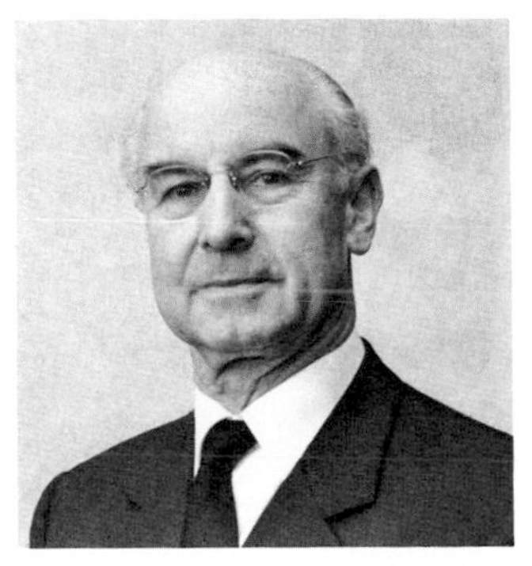

IT IS OFTEN STATED in the literature that LSD was discovered by chance. The following account will show that LSD was not the fruit of a chance discovery, but the outcome of a more complex process that had its beginnings in a definite concept, and was followed up by appropriate experiments, during the course of which a chance observation served to trigger off a planned investigation, which then led to the actual discovery. Such a train of events often underlies what is said to be a chance discovery.

I prepared lysergic acid diethylamide for the first time in 1938 as part of a systematic chemical and pharmacological investigation of partially synthetic amides of lysergic acid in the Sandoz pharmaceutical-chemical research laboratories in Basle, headed at that time by Professor Arthur Stoll. Lysergic acid is the characteristic nucleus of the alkaloids of ergot and can be obtained by alkaline

* Director of Research, Department of Natural Products, Sandoz Ltd., Basel, Switzerland.

hydrolysis of these alkaloids. Using a newly developed procedure, one had proved it possible to combine lysergic acid with amines in peptide linkage. In this way, the specific oxytocic principle of ergot, namely Ergometrine, known in this country as ergonovine, was produced. This was the first partial synthesis of a natural ergot alkaloid, and by modifying the alkanolamine side chain of Ergometrine a new synthetic derivative, which we named Methergine, was obtained. In its pharmacological properties Methergine proved to be superior to the natural alkaloid, and today it is used throughout the world in obstetrics for the arrest of hemorrhage. Although interest centered mainly on oxytocic and hemostatic activity in these investigations, the new method of synthesis was also employed to prepare amides of lysergic acid, which, on the basis of their chemical structure, might be expected to possess different pharmacological properties. Thus among other compounds, I synthesized the diethylamide of lysergic acid with the intention of obtaining an analeptic. This compound might have been expected to possess analeptic properties because of its structural relationship with the well-known circulatory stimulant nikethamide.

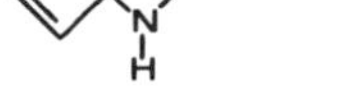

Ergometrine ($R = CH_3$)
Methergine® ($R = CH_2CH_3$)

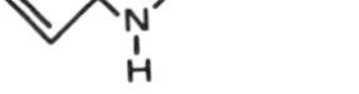

Lysergic acid diethylamide
LSD

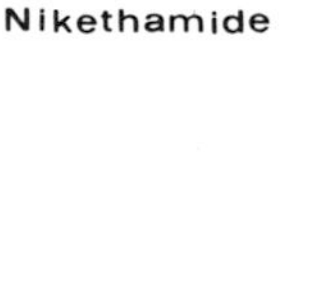

Nikethamide

A number of pharmacological experiments were carried out by Professor Ernst Rothlin with this new compound, which was given the laboratory code name LSD-25 because it was the twenty-fifth compound of the lysergic acid amide series. These experiments revealed a fairly marked uterotonic action, not unexpected in view of the close chemical relationship between LSD and the oxytocic drugs Ergometrine and Methergine. In addition, marked excitation was observed in some of the animals. Work on LSD then fell into abeyance for a number of years.

Because I had the feeling that it would be worth while to carry out more profound studies with this compound, I prepared a fresh quantity of LSD in 1943. In the course of this work an accidental observation led me to carry out a planned self-experiment with this compound. The following is an extract of my report on these experiments, dated April 22, 1943, and addressed to the Head of the Pharmaceutical Department, Professor Stoll.

> Last Friday, April 16, 1943, I was forced to stop my work in the laboratory in the middle of the afternoon and to go home, as I was seized by a peculiar restlessness associated with a sensation of mild dizziness. On arriving home, I lay down and sank into a kind of drunkenness which was not unpleasant and which was characterized by extreme activity of imagination. As I lay in a dazed condition with my eyes closed (I experienced daylight as disagreeably bright) there surged upon me an uninterrupted stream of fantastic images of extraordinary plasticity and vividness and accompanied by an intense, kaleidoscope-like play of colors. This condition gradually passed off after about two hours.

The nature and the course of this extraordinary disturbance raised my suspicions that some exogenic intoxication may have been involved and that the lysergic acid diethylamide with which I had been working that afternoon could have been responsible. I had separated the two isomeric forms that are formed by this synthesis, namely lysergic diethylamide and isolysergic acid diethylamide and prepared the crystalline water soluble salt of lysergic acid diethylamide with tartaric acid. However, I could not imagine how this compound could have accidentally found its way into my body in a sufficient quantity to produce such phenomena. Moreover, the nature of the symptoms did not tally with those previously associated with ergot poisoning. In order to get to the root of the matter, I decided to conduct some experiments on myself with the substance in question. I started with the lowest dose that might be expected to have any effect, i.e., 0.25 mg LSD. The notes in my laboratory journal read as follows:

> April 19, 1943: Preparation of an 0.5% aqueous solution of d-lysergic acid diethylamide tartrate.
> 4:20 P.M.: 0.5 cc (0.25 mg LSD) ingested orally. The solution is tasteless.
> 4:50 P.M.: no trace of any effect.
> 5:00 P.M.: slight dizziness, unrest, difficulty in concentration, visual disturbances, marked desire to laugh . . .

At this point the laboratory notes are discontinued: The last words were written only with great difficulty. I asked my laboratory assistant to accompany me home as I believed that I should have a repetition of the disturbance of the previous Friday. While we were cycling home, however, it became clear that the symptoms were much stronger than the first time. I had great difficulty in speaking coherently, my field of vision swayed before me, and objects appeared distorted like images in curved mirrors. I had the impression of being unable to move from the spot, although my assistant told me afterwards that we had cycled at a good pace. . . . Once I was at home the physician was called.

> By the time the doctor arrived, the peak of the crisis had already passed. As far as I remember, the following were the most outstanding symptoms: vertigo, visual disturbances; the faces of those around me appeared as grotesque, colored masks; marked motoric unrest, alternating with paralysis; an intermittent heavy feeling in the head, limbs and the entire body, as if they were filled with lead; dry, constricted sensation in the throat; feeling of choking; clear recognition of my condition, in which state I sometimes observed, in the manner of an independent, neutral observer, that I shouted half insanely or babbled incoherent words. Occasionally I felt as if I were out of my body.
>
> The doctor found a rather weak pulse but an otherwise normal circulation. . . . Six hours after ingestion of the LSD my condition had already improved considerably. Only the visual disturbances were still pronounced. Everything seemed to sway and the proportions were distorted like the reflections in the surface of moving water. Moreover, all objects appeared in unpleasant, constantly changing colors, the predominant shades being sickly green and blue. When I closed my eyes, an unending series of colorful, very realistic and fantastic images surged in upon me. A remarkable feature was the manner in which all acoustic perceptions (e.g., the noise of a passing car) were transformed into optical effects, every sound evoking a corresponding colored hallucination constantly changing in shape and color like pictures in a kaleidoscope. At about one o'clock I fell asleep and awoke next morning feeling perfectly well.

This was the first planned experiment with LSD and a rather dramatic one. Subsequent experiments on volunteer colleagues of the Sandoz research laboratories confirmed the extraordinary activity of LSD on the human psyche. These showed that the effective oral dose of LSD in human beings is 0.03 mg to 0.05 mg. In spite of my caution, I had chosen for my first experiment five times the average effective dose. LSD is by far the most active and most specific hallucinogen. It is about 5,000 to 10,000 times more active than mescaline, which produces qualitatively nearly the same symptoms. The extremely high potency of LSD is not just a curiosity; it is in many respects of the greatest scientific interest. For example, it lent support to the hypothesis that certain mental illnesses that were supposed until then to be of purely psychic nature had a biochemical cause because it now seemed feasible that undetectable traces of a psychoactive substance produced by the body itself might produce psychic disturbances.

LSD was unique with regard to its extremely high hallucinogenic potency. But it was not new with regard to the quality of its hallucinogenic property. As already mentioned, it produces qualitatively the same psychic effects as mescaline, a hallucinogen known long before LSD, mescaline being the active principle of one of the ancient magic plants of Mexico. Hallucinogenic drugs were of great importance in the old Indian cultures of Central America. The Spanish chroniclers and naturalists who came to the country soon after the conquest of Mexico by Cortes mentioned in their writings a great number of plants with psychic effects. These plants were unknown in the Old World and were used by the Indians both in their medical practices and in their religious ceremonies. The cultic use and divine worship paid to many of these drugs met with the disapproval of the Christian missionaries, who attempted by any means possible to liberate the Indians from this "devilry." They were only partially successful, however, in this respect. The native population secretly continued to use the drugs, which they considered to be holy even after they had been converted to Christianity.

Three main magic plants were used by the Aztecs and neighboring tribes in their religious ceremonies and in their medical practices, which were strongly influenced by magical concepts; these drugs are still used today for the same purpose by the witch doctors in remote districts of Mexico. They are:

1/ peyotl, a cactus species,
2/ teonanacatl, certain foliate mushrooms, and
3/ ololiuqui, the seeds of certain bindweeds.

The first magic plant to be studied scientifically was peyotl, also named peyote; this was under investigation as early as at the turn of the century. The history of peyotl, its ancient cultic use by the Indians of Central America and its present use, as well as the psychic effects on human beings, were first described by Louis Lewin, the brilliant pharmacologist and toxicologist, in his classic monograph entitled *Phantasticka.*[1]

Lewin established the basis for psychotomimetic research by this standard publication in which the psychotomimetics or hallucinogens, named by him *Phantastika,* were characterized and grouped for the first time in an independent group within the psychopharmaceutical drugs. The peyotl cactus was named by the botanist Hennings *Anhalonium lewinii* in honor of Lewin. Louis Lewin and Arthur Heffter, who isolated the alkaloid mescaline in 1896 from the cactus, deserve a place of honor in the history of psychopharmacological psychotomimetic research.[2] In 1919, Ernst Späth in Vienna succeeded in elucidating the chemical structure of mescaline and in synthesizing this alkaloid.[3]

Mescaline made it possible for the first time to investigate the phenomenon of hallucinogenic effects from a scientific, pharmacological, and clinical aspect using a pure chemical compound. The results of this first period of psychopharmacological investigations in the nineteen twenties were published in the classical monograph *Der Meskalinrausch* by K. Beringer.[4] However, in the years to follow, interest in hallucinogenic research faded. Not until the nineteen forties with the discovery of LSD did this line of research receive a new impetus leading to an upsurge of interest that has lasted until the present time.

Our preoccupation with LSD was the reason why the second magic drug of Mexico, teonanacatl, which means "sacred mushroom," was submitted to our laboratory for a chemical analysis. The use and worship of teonanacatl by the Indians of Central America must be very ancient. In Guatemala, "mushroom stones" have been found the oldest specimens of which are over three thousand years old.

Although the mushroom cult is very old, our knowledge of it is very recent. For some centuries the reports in the old chronicles were given surprisingly little attention, probably because they were regarded as extravagances of a superstitious age. It was not until 1936 to 1938 that American investigators, i.e., Weitlander, Reko, Johnson and Schultes, ascertained that mushrooms were still being eaten for magical purposes by the natives in certain remote dis-

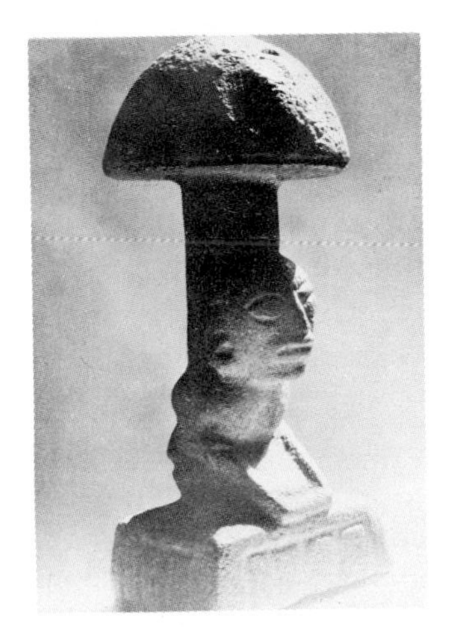

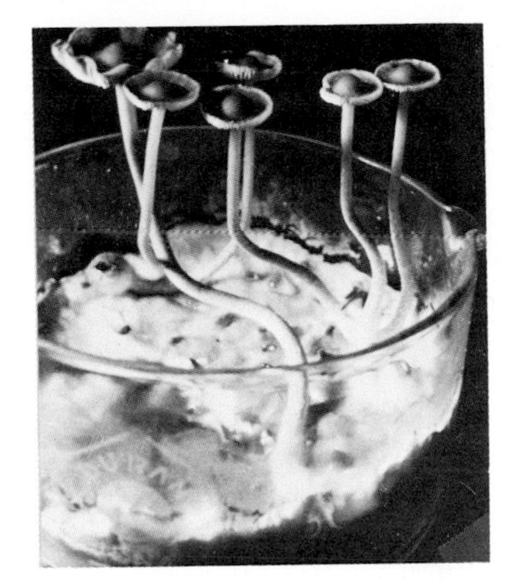

FIG. 1. Mushroom stone. FIG. 2. *Psilocybe mexicana Heim.*

tricts of southern Mexico. Systematic studies of the mushroom cult in its present form were later made by the amateur investigators R. Gordon Wasson and his wife. In the summer of 1955, Wasson was able for the first time to take active part in a secret nocturnal ceremony in Huautla de Jimenez Province of Oaxaca, and was probably the first white man to ingest the holy mushrooms. On a later expedition in 1956, Wasson was accompanied by the mycologist Roger Heim, director of the Laboratoire de Cryptogamie du Museum National d'Histoire Naturelle in Paris. Heim succeeded in identifying the sacred mushrooms and classifying them botanically. They belong to the family of Strophariaceae, principally to the genus *Psilocybe,* though one species belongs to the genus *Stropharia* and another to the genus *Conocybe.* Artificial cultivation in the laboratory provided a good yield of especially one of these sacred mushrooms, namely, *Psilocybe mexicana Heim.*

After unsuccessful attempts in Paris to isolate the active principles, Professor Heim sent the mushrooms to the Sandoz Research Laboratories in Basle, believing that our experience with LSD would enable us to solve this problem. In a sense, therefore, LSD brought the sacred mushrooms to our laboratory.

In the first phase of our isolation studies, we tried to evaluate the extracts by testing them on animals, observing pupillary reaction and piloerection in mice and general behavior in dogs. But the results were not clear-cut and led to discrepancies in the evaluation of the various extract fractions. After most of the very rare and valuable mushroom material had been used for animal testing without definite results, there was some doubt whether the mushrooms cultivated and dried in Paris were still active at all. In order to settle this fundamental point, I decided to test them on myself. I ate 32 dried specimens of *Psilocybe mexicana* weighing 2.4 g, corresponding to a medium dose by Indian standards. I shall describe my experience by reading the English translation of my original published report of that experiment:

> Thirty minutes after my taking the mushrooms, the exterior world began to undergo a strange transformation. Everything assumed a Mexican character. As I was perfectly well aware that my knowledge of the Mexican origin of the mushroom would lead me to imagine only Mexican scenery, I tried deliberately to look on my environment as I knew it normally. But all voluntary efforts to look at things in their customary forms and colors proved ineffective. Whether my eyes were closed or open, I saw only Mexican motifs and colors. When the doctor supervising the experiment bent over me to check my blood pressure, he was transformed into an Aztec priest and I would not have been astonished if he had drawn an obsidian knife. In spite of the seriousness of the situation, it amused me to see how the Germanic face of my colleague had acquired a purely Indian expression. At the peak of the intoxication, about 1½ hours after ingestion of the mushrooms, the rush of interior pictures, mostly abstract motifs rapidly changing in shape and color, reached such an alarming degree that I feared that I would be torn into this whirlpool of form and color and would dissolve. After about six hours the dream came to an end. Subjectively, I had no idea how long this condition had lasted. I felt my return to everyday reality to be a happy return from a strange, fantastic but quite real world to an old and familiar home.

This personal study showed that the negative results of the tests in animals were due not to the mushroom material but to the ani-

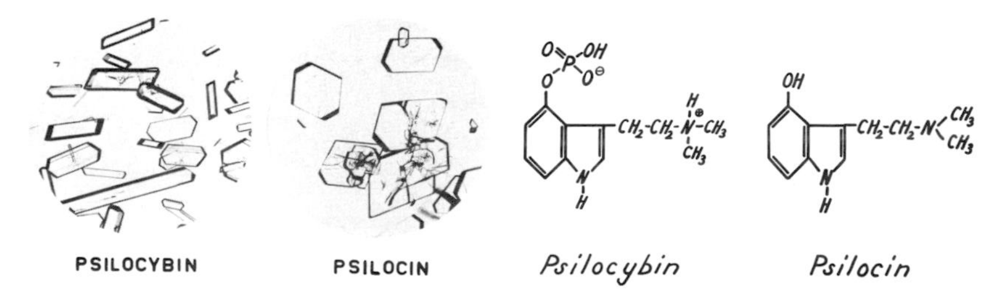

FIG. 3. Crystals of psilocybin and psilocin, and formulas.

mals used and that human beings provide a more sensitive index of substances with psychic effects than animals. With the aid of this reliable test in human beings, it was then possible to extract the active principles from the mushroom and to purify and crystallize them. The main active component was named psilocybin, and an accompanying alkaloid, usually present only in small amounts, named psilocin.

The elucidation of their structures showed that these were a novel type of indole derivatives. Psilocybin is the first and only hitherto known natural indole compound that contains a phosphoric acid radical. Furthermore, psilocin and psilocybin were the first indole alkaloids with a free or phosphorylated hydroxyl group at the position 4 of the indole ring system, all the other numerous indole alkaloids bearing hydroxyl groups at the positions 5, 6 or 7.

The final proof of the correctness of the proposed structures was provided by the total synthesis of psilocin and psilocybin. The synthetic production of psilocybin and psilocin is now more economical than obtaining them from the mushrooms. My colleagues

OH, CH_3, NO_2 — 4 steps → $OCH_2C_6H_5$ (indole, N–H) — 1) $(COCl)_2$ 2) $HN(CH_3)_2$ → $OCH_2C_6H_5$, $CO{-}CO{-}N(CH_3)_2$

1) $LiAlH_4$ 2) Pd/H_2 → OH, $CH_2{-}CH_2{-}N(CH_3)_2$

$O{=}P(OCH_2C_6H_5)_2Cl$ → $O{=}P(OCH_2C_6H_5)_2{-}O$, $CH_2{-}CH_2{-}N(CH_3)_2$

Pd/H_2 → $O{=}P(OH)(O^{(-)}){-}O$, $CH_2{-}CH_2{-}N^{(+)}H(CH_3)_2$

Psilocybin

who participated in these investigations were: Dr. Arthur Brack, Dr. Albert Frey, Dr. Hans Kobel, Dr. Hans Ott, Dr. Theodor Petrzilka and Dr. Franz Troxler.[5]

A review of the historical, ethnological, botanical and chemical aspects of the hallucinogenic Mexican mushrooms is presented in the beautiful volume, *Les champignons hallucinogènes*, by Roger Heim and R. Gordon Wasson, edited by the Museum National d'Histoire Naturelle in Paris.[6] An average human oral dose of psilocybin is 6 mg to 10 mg. Psilocin possesses similar activity. This means that psilocybin and psilocin are about 100 times more active than mescaline and about 100 times less active than LSD. But there is no significant difference between the two compounds in quality of hallucinogenic activity. The development of cross-tolerance between LSD and psilocybin lends support to the view that these two drugs cause psychic disturbances by acting on some common mechanism, or on mechanisms acting through a common final pathway.

When I was in Mexico on an expedition with my friend Gordon Wasson in 1963, in search of a hallucinogenic plant, we also visited the famous curandera Maria Sabina in Huautla de Jimenez. We were invited to attend a nocturnal mushroom ceremony in her hut, but as it was late in the year and no more mushrooms were available, I supplied her with pills containing synthetic psilocybin. She took a rather strong dose corresponding to the number of mushrooms she usually ingests. It was a gala performance assisted by a number of people of Maria Sabina's clan. At dawn when we left the hut, our Mazateca interpreter told us that Maria Sabina had said there was no difference between the pills and the mushrooms. This was a final proof that our synthetic psilocybin was identical in every respect with the natural product.

That was the story of the second magic Mexican drug of teonanacatl. But there was still the riddle of ololiuqui, the third magic Mexican drug. Ololiuqui is the Aztec name for the seeds of certain convolvulaceous plants that since prehispanic times have been used by the Aztecs and related tribes in their religious ceremonies and magic medicinal practices in the same way as the sacred mushrooms and the cactus peyotl. Ololiuqui is still used in our day by such tribes as the Zapotecs, Chinantecs, Mazatecs, and Mixtecs, who live in the remote mountains of southern Mexico in comparative isolation, little influenced by Christianity. An excellent review of the historical, ethnological and botanical aspects of the ololiuqui question was given in 1941 by R. Evans Schultes of the Botanical Museum at Harvard, in his monograph, *A Contribution to our Knowledge of Rivea corymbosa. The Narcotic Ololiuqui of the Aztecs.*[7]

De OLILIVHQVI, ſeu planta orbicularium foliorum. Cap. XIV.

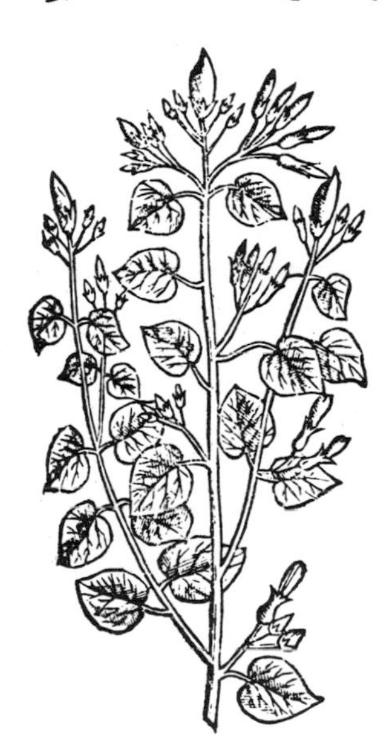

OLILIVHQVI, quam *Coaxihuitl*, ſeu herbam Serpentis alij vocant, volubilis herba eſt, folia viridia ferens, tenuia, cordis figura. caules teretes, virides, tenueſq;. flores albos, & longiuſculos. ſemen rotundum ſimile Coriandro, vnde nomen. radices fibris ſimiles. calida quarto ordine planta eſt. luem Gallicam curat. dolores è frigore ortos ſedat. flatum, ac præter naturam tumores diſcutit. puluis reſina mixtus pellit frigus. luxatis aut fractis oſſibus, & lumbis fœminarum laxis, aucto robore mirum auxiliatur in modum. Seminis etiam eſt vſus in medicina, quod tritum, ac deuoratum, illitumq; capiti, & fronti, cum lacte & *Chilli*, fertur morbis oculorum mederi. deuoratum verò, venerem excitat. Acri eſt ſapore, & temperie, veluti & planta eius, impensè calida. Indorum ſacrifici cum videri volebant verſari cum Superis, ac reſpōſa accipere ab eis, ea veſcebātur planta, vt deſiperent, milleq; phantaſmata, & dæmonū obuerſātium effigies circumſpectarent. qua in re Solano maniaco Dioſcoridis ſimilis fortaſſe alicui videri poſſit.

The first description and illustration of ololiuqui was published by Francisco Hernandez, a Spanish physician, who between 1570 and 1575 carried out extensive research on the flora and fauna of Mexico for Philip II. In his famous *Rerum Medicarum Novae Hispaniae Thesaurus, seu Plantarium, Animalium, Mineralium Mexicanorum Historia,* which appeared in 1651 in Rome, Hernandez described ololiuqui under the heading "De Oliliuhqui, seu planta orbicularium foliorum." An extract of the translation of the 1651 Latin version reads as follows:

> Oliliuhqui, which some call coaxihuitl, or snake plant, is a twining herb with thin, green cordate leaves, slender, green terete stems and long white flowers. The seed is round and very like coriander. . . . Formerly, when the priests wished to commune with their gods and to receive a message from them, they ate this plant to induce a delirium. A thousand visions and satanic hallucinations appeared to them. . . .

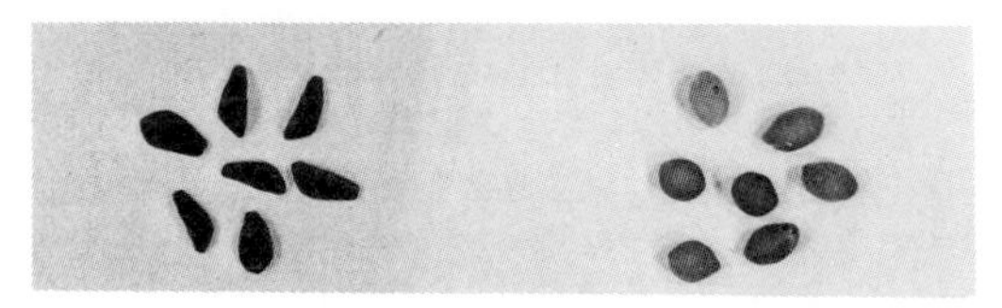

FIG. 5. Seeds of *Rivea corymbosa* and *Ipomoea tricolor.*

The only report of chemical studies on the seeds of *Rivea corymbosa* mentioned in Schultes' review on ololiuqui is that of the pharmacologist Santesson in Stockholm in 1937. He was, however, unsuccessful in isolating definite crystalline compounds. Alcoholic extracts produced a kind of narcosis or partial narcosis in frogs and mice.

In 1955, the Canadian psychiatrist Osmond conducted a series of experiments on himself.[8] After taking 60 to 100 Rivea seeds he passed into a state of apathy and listlessness accompanied by increased visual sensitivity. After about four hours, there followed a period in which he had a relaxed feeling of well-being that lasted for a rather longer time. In contrast to these results, Kinross-Wright in 1958 published experiments performed on eight male volunteers who had taken doses of up to 125 seeds without any ascertainable effect.[9]

After the chemical investigations of the sacred Mexican mushrooms had been successfully brought to a close, I decided to tackle the problem of the third Mexican magic drug, ololiuqui. Through the help of R. G. Wasson, I was able to obtain authentic ololiuqui from a Zapotec Indian near Oaxaca in southern Mexico. One sample consisted of brown seeds, which proved on botanical classification to stem from *Rivea corymbosa.* The black seeds of the second sample were identical with those of *Ipomoea violacea L.* (syn. *Ipomoea tricolor CAV.*). These black seeds, called "badoh negro," are used especially in the region of the Zapotecs, in conjunction with, or instead of "Badoh," the brown seeds of *Rivea corymbosa.*

The chemical analysis of the ololiuqui seeds gave a quite surprising result. The psychotomimetic principles that we isolated proved to be lysergic acid derivatives, lysergic acid amides and other ergot alkaloids.[10] Thus in this strange Mexican drug we met with old friends, since lysergic acid derivatives and ergot alkaloids had been favorite subjects of research in our laboratory since the time I had first synthesized LSD in the nineteen-thirties.

The main constituents of ololiuqui, i.e., the seeds of *Rivea corym-*

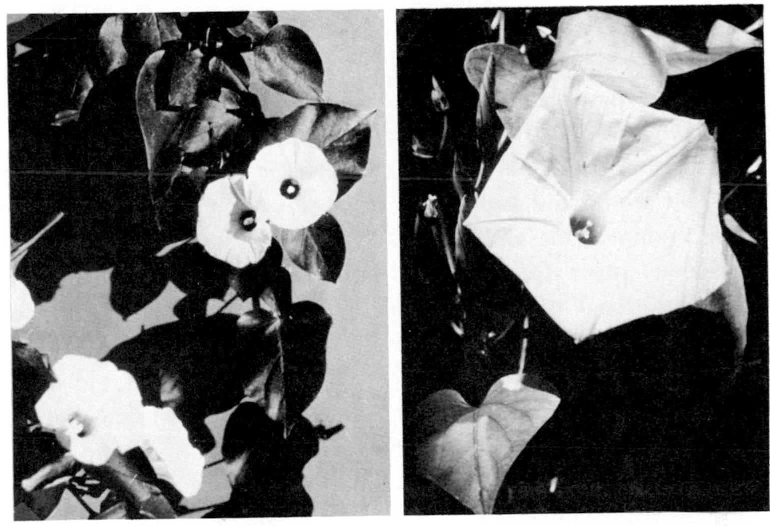

FIG. 6. Flowering plants of *Rivea corymbosa* and *Ipomoea tricolor.*

bosa, are lysergic acid amide and lysergic acid 1-hydroxyethylamide. The active constituents of ololiuqui are very closely related to LSD. The only difference between the main constituent of ololiuqui, lysergic acid amide, and LSD is that the two hydrogen atoms of the amide are replaced by two ethyl radicals. It is a very

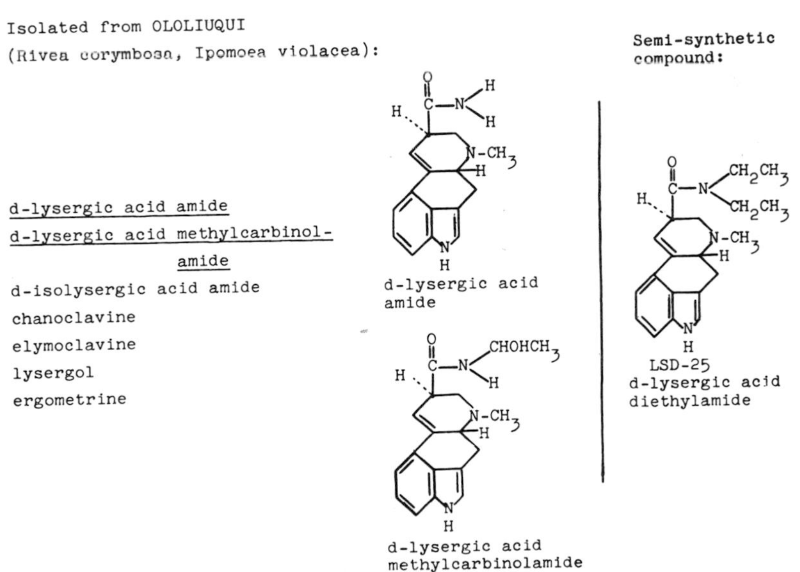

FIG. 7. Structural relation between active principles of ololiuqui and LSD-25.

significant one with regard to the psychotomimetic activity. The ololiuqui principle, lysergic acid amide, is much less active than lysergic acid diethylamide (LSD), and provokes psychic symptoms qualitatively different from those of LSD, as will be shown later.

Furthermore, the following minor alkaloids were isolated: isolysergic acid amide and isolysergic acid 1-hydroxyethylamide, chanoclavin, elymoclavine and lysergol. The seeds of the related convolvulaceous plant *Ipomoea violacea* yielded the same alkaloids with the difference that ergometrine was present instead of lysergol. The occurrence of ergot alkaloids in higher plants, in the phanerogamic family Convolvulaceae was quite unexpected and is of particular interest from the phytochemical point of view because lysergic acid alkaloids had hitherto been isolated only from genera of lower fungi: Claviceps, Penicillium and Rhizopus. Lysergic acid amide, the main component of ololiuqui, had been tested pharmacologically and clinically under the experimental drug designation LA-111 during the course of our investigations on LSD and related compounds long before it was known to be a natural component of a magic Mexican drug. Self-experiment and comparative systematic clinical investigations with lysergic acid amide (laboratory code name: LA-111) revealed psychotomimetic effects significantly different from those of lysergic acid diethylamide (LSD-25). The symptoms after oral ingestion of 1 mg to 2 mg of LA-111 were: indifference, decrease of psychomotor activity, tiredness, feeling of sinking into nothingness, and desire to sleep. Isolysergic amide produces similar symptoms. After taking 2.0 mg of isolysergic amide orally, I experienced tiredness, apathy, a feeling of mental emptiness and of the unreality and complete meaninglessness of the outside world.[11] These comparative experiments showed that the psychotomimetic constituents of ololiuqui are 20 to 40 times less active than LSD and that the general picture of activity is characterized by a pronounced depressive and narcotic component.

I now come to the last section of my chapter; here I shall discuss very briefly some common features in the chemical structure of the hallucinogens I have discussed. The comparison of these structures reveals an interesting relationship with the structures of important neurohumoral substances. This is certainly no mere coincidence, but of major importance.

Mescaline, being a phenylethylamine derivative, is structurally

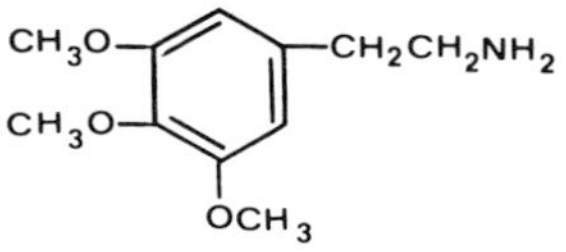

Mescaline

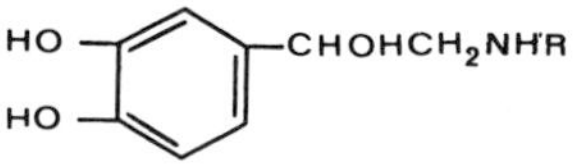

R = H : Norepinephrine
R = CH_3 : Epinephrine

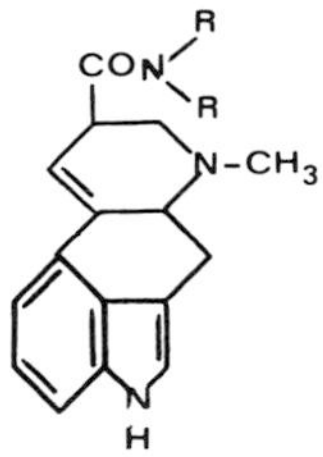

R = H : Lysergic acid amide (Ololiuqui)
R = C_2H_5 : LSD

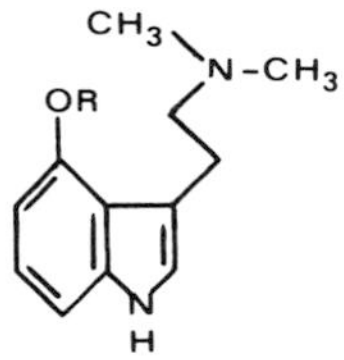

R = PO_3H_2 : Psilocybin
R = H : Psilocin

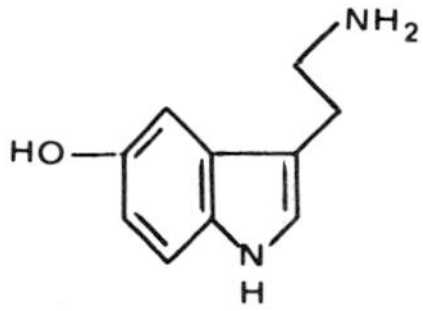

Serotonin

related to the neurohumoral transmitters norepinephrine and epinephrine. LSD, and the constituents of ololiuqui as well as the active principles of the hallucinogenic mushrooms psilocybin and psilocin, are indoles, more precisely tryptamine derivates, like the neurohumoral factor serotonin. Because of this structural relationship between the hallucinogens and norepinephrine and serotonin, it is probable that the psychotomimetic activity is due to an interaction between these substances in the metabolism of the central nervous system. Investigation of the relationships between endogenous neurohumoral factors and hallucinogens is a rewarding facet of psychopharmacological research.

As I am a chemist, I have mainly discussed the chemical, phytochemical and historical aspects of the discovery of LSD and the investigation of naturally occurring hallucinogens. Needless to say, this audience attaches primary importance to the pharmacological and clinical effects, which make LSD and the other specific hallucinogens a valuable tool in experimental psychiatry and a valuable drug aid in psychoanalysis and psychotherapy. Another aspect of the hallucinogens and especially of LSD with enormous social impact is of course the paramedical use and the misuse of these substances. But this very complex problem would provide material for a special lecture, or indeed for a series of such lectures.

The aim of my chapter is to describe an unusual cycle of chemical research, full of coincidences, a kind of magic circle, which started with the synthesis of various lysergic acid amides and the discovery of the extraordinary psychotomimetic potency of lysergic acid diethylamide (LSD), which led to the investigation of the sacred Mexican mushrooms, the isolation of psilocybin, and ended with ololiuqui, where lysergic acid amides were again encountered, thus closing the magic circle.

REFERENCES

1. Lewin, L.: Phantastika, Berlin, Georg Stilke, 1924. Second enlarged edition published in 1927. The first English edition appeared in 1931. A new impression 1964: Phantastica, Narcotic and Stimulating Drugs, Their Use and Abuse, London, Routledge and Kegan Paul, 1964.
2. Heffter, A.: Ber *29*:216, 1896.
3. Späth, E.: Monatsh *40*:129, 1919.
4. Beringer, K.: Der Meskalinrausch, Berlin, Springer, 1927.
5. Hofmann, A., *et al.*: Helv Chim Acta *42*:1557, 1959.
6. Heim, R., and Wasson, R. G.: Les Champignons hallucinogènes du Mexique, ed. du Muséum national d'Histoire Naturelle, Paris, 1958.
7. Schultes, R. E.: A Contribution to Our Knowledge of Rivea Corymbosa: The Narcotic Ololiuqui of the Aztecs, Botanical Museum, Harvard Univ, Cambridge (Mass), 1941.
8. Osmond, H.: J Ment Sci *101*:526, 1955.
9. Kinross-Wright, V. J.: *In* Bradley, P. B., Deniker, P., and Raduoco-Thomas C., eds.: Neuro-Psychopharmacology, Amsterdam, Elsevier, 1959, p. 453.
10. Hofmann, A.: Planta Med *9*:354, 1961.
11. ——: Botan Museum Leaflets, Harvard Univ *20*:194, 1963.

CHAPTER

8

Indoklon—A Fluorinated Ether Convulsant

JOHN C. KRANTZ, JR., PHD *

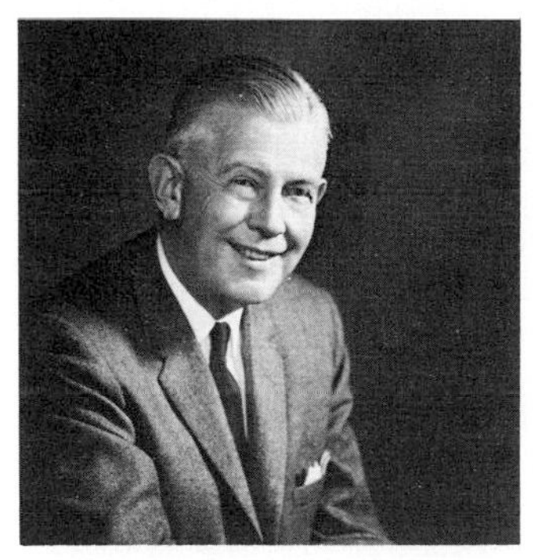

THAT THE LIVING CELL can become the site of consciousness is one of the most intriguing, yet baffling, problems in biology. Equally mystifying is that one can evoke a hiatus or discontinuity in consciousness, called surgical anesthesia, with a series of chemically unrelated compounds. Although these agents enter and leave the brain without undergoing chemical change, the central nervous system (CNS) is exquisitely sensitive to their chemical configurations. For example, let us consider the three cyclic hydrocarbons, cyclopropane, cyclobutane and cyclopentane:

				CH_2	
CH_2		H_2C	CH_2	H_2C	CH_2
H_2C	CH_2	H_2C	CH_2	H_2C	CH_2
cyclopropane		cyclobutane		cyclopentane	

Cyclobutane, like cyclopropane, is an excellent anesthetic and resembles cyclopropane in many of its characteristics. One might expect

* Director of Pharmacologic Research, Maryland Psychiatric Research Center, Baltimore.

cyclopentane to exhibit a similar pharmacologic response. Cyclopentane, however, evokes mild convulsive seizures in laboratory animals.

The modern era of fluorinated anesthetics is recent in origin, dating back to the early 1950s.[1] The element fluorine was discovered by Ampère in France in 1810. It was named fluorine after calcium fluoride CaF_2, which is used as a flux (meaning to make fluid upon heating). Fluorine is the most active of all the nonmetallic elements. As an acceptor of electrons, its avidity for electrons far exceeds that of oxygen. Alcohol, cork, turpentine and other organic substances ignite spontaneously in an atmosphere of fluorine. Even the noble gas xenon unites with fluorine to form XeF_4. The first organic fluoride prepared was CF_4, which was synthesized accidentally in an unsuccessful attempt to isolate elemental fluorine in a carbon vessel. During the '30s and '40s there were a few sporadic attempts to prepare and study the pharmacologic properties of the fluorinated hydrocarbons. The most outstanding and comprehensive of these studies was conducted by Robbins in 1946.[2]

Our interest in the fluorinated ethers and hydrocarbons originated in the late '40s.[3] During World War II, new methods of fluorination had been developed, and many fluorinated compounds that at one time were laboratory curiosities were now commercially available. Our aims were twofold: *1/* to determine the effect of fluorination on anesthetic properties and *2/* to eliminate the fire hazard involved in the use of volatile anesthetics. These studies resulted in the introduction of trifluoroethyl vinyl ether (Fluoromar) into clinical anesthesia. In the spring of 1953, I anesthetized Dr. Max Sadove with Fluoromar. He was the first man on this planet to be anesthetized with a fluorinated anesthetic, and this started the fluorine revolution in anesthesia.

One might fittingly ask What are the properties conferred upon a hydrocarbon or an ether that make them so desirable as anesthetics? First, the introduction of a fluorine atom into a hydrocarbon molecule markedly reduces the boiling point and permits certain chlorinated hydrocarbons and ethers to be used that would otherwise be unavailable. For example, *CH_3Cl boils at –23°C, but $CF_3.Cl$ boils at –82°C*. A liquid boils when its molecules possess sufficient kinetic energy to overcome the attractive force of its molecules. The intramolecular force of fluorinated molecules is relatively great, and the intermolecular force is relatively small. Therefore, the heat energy required for vaporization is less than that required by other halogenated hydrocarbons in which the converse inter- and intra-molecular forces prevail.

Following the principle that all drugs available are subject to improvement, we began to study the analogs and homologs of Fluoromar. In the summer of 1956, we studied hexafluorodiethyl ether $CF_3.CH_2\text{-}O\text{-}CH_2.CF_3$, which we expected to be an anesthetic less potent than Fluoromar. Much to our surprise, this agent was not an anesthetic, but evoked marked CNS stimulation and convulsive seizures. It is the function of the pharmacologist to project the action of a compound on laboratory animals to its possible use in the treatment of disease in man. The possible use of hexafluorodiethyl ether (Indoklon) as a substitute for electroshock therapy (ECT) in the treatment of the mentally ill suggested itself to our research team.

Accordingly, through many months of experiments on a variety of laboratory animals, Indoklon was used to induce convulsive seizures upon the inhalation of its vapor. Not any species of laboratory animals failed to convulse upon exposure to Indoklon vapor in concentrations as low as 35 parts per million of inspired air. Immediately on the removal of Indoklon, the seizure ceased. Batteries of organ functional tests and pathologic investigations revealed no residual harmful effect of the exposure to Indoklon.[4]

The exposure of the first patient to Indoklon seizures involved a problem in medical ethics. Everyone is a candidate for anesthesia. Only certain persons who are mentally ill are subject to ECT. It was my opinion that we had the moral right to try Indoklon on such patients only. Accordingly, four mentally ill patients for whom electroshock was indicated were subjected by the author on September 20, 1956, to the inhalation of Indoklon. The agent was placed in a plastic inhaler of the type used for the administration of nasal decongestants. After one to three minutes inhalation, classic tonic grand mal type seizures followed that lasted for several minutes. Recovery was uneventful. In cooperation with Dr. Albert A. Kurland, an extensive investigation followed at Spring Grove State Hospital. The treatment appeared tantamount to that of electroshock, with marked patient preference. Frequently, patients who did not improve under ECT improved when Indoklon therapy was substituted.

One of the interesting observations made in this study resulted from our experiments with an isomer of Indoklon. The relationship of the two molecules is shown in the formulas:

$CF_3 \cdot CH_2\text{-}O\text{-}CH_2 \cdot CF_3$

Indoklon

$$\begin{matrix} CF_3 \\ CF_3 \end{matrix} CH\text{-}O\text{-}CH_3$$

Isoindoklon

Isoindoklon, unlike Indoklon, is an anesthetic with potency somewhat greater than that of diethyl ether. The actions of the two isomers antagonized each other on laboratory animals. This antagonism is illustrated in Table 1.

TABLE 1. *Effect of Indoklon and Isoindoklon on Mice* *

VOL. % ISO.	VOL. % INDO.	NUMBER CONVULSIONS	TIME OF ONSET OF SEIZURE SEC.	NUMBER DEATHS
0.00	0.25	8	30	1
0.63	0.25	1	300	0
1.25	0.25	0	—	0
0.00	0.50	10	5	9
0.63	0.50	9	40	0
1.25	0.50	2	45	0
2.50	0.50	0	—	0

* 10 mice in each group exposed for 10 min.

The data in Table 1 show that the effect of fatal concentrations of Indoklon vapor is nullified by appropriate concentrations of the vapor of isoindoklon. Furthermore, it was observed that the behavior of mice exposed to a mixture of 1.25 vol % of Isoindoklon and 0.25 vol % of Indoklon was not affected in any way that could be differentiated from normal mice. We termed this condition "balanced state," which could be maintained for long time periods.

We conducted many studies designed to detect a difference between these two isomers that in some manner might suggest a reason for this definitive antagonism of activity of these two isomers. Table 2 shows a comparison of these properties.

From Table 2, the only difference between the measurements that may have significance is that of the O/W coefficient.[5] This is approximately four times greater for the anesthetic than for Indoklon, the convulsant.

This observation and other studies conducted by us on the effect

TABLE 2. *Physicochemical Measurements*

	INDOKLON	ISOINDOKLON
Liquid molar vol. 37°ml/mole	132	137
$\Delta H_v 37°K$ cal/mole	6.75	6.49
Dipole moment	2.4	2.9
Interfacial tension	19.2 dynes/cm	18.5
Viscosity	0.66	0.51 (H_2O = 1)
Surface tension saturated aqueous solution	72 dynes/cm	72
Solubility in water	0.2 vol. %	0.8
Oil/water coefficient	66 ± 5	200 ± 5

of fluoroform CHF_3 and Reon E-1 (an inactive fluorinated ether) led us to the following concept of the action of these agents. There are two receptor sites in the brain: one possessing a configuration into which the molecule of the convulsive precisely fits; the other presenting a matrix to which the molecule of the anesthetic may be absorbed with exactness of fit. Nevertheless, there is, as one might expect, some overlapping on the respective receptor sites, as Indoklon evokes facets of the anesthetic syndrome, and anesthetics elicit excitation characteristic of the convulsives.

In our study of the mechanism of action of Indoklon, we have observed that the compound releases acetylcholine from its binding sites in the brain.[6] This is indicative of intensified neuronal transmission. Furthermore, it promotes the retention of cerebral intracellular sodium and the release of potassium. The anticonvulsive drug diphenylhydantoin sodium reverses this type of ionic exchange, and it is proposed that its anticonvulsive action is due, at least in part, to the release of intracellular sodium. It has been demonstrated that human epileptogenic foci are relatively high in sodium content and low in potassium.

Let us return now to the clinical use of Indoklon. Early in our studies with Indoklon at Spring Grove State Hospital, the distinguished psychiatrist Dr. Lothar Kalinowsky, father of electroshock therapy in America, visited the treatment room to witness the use of Indoklon. He appeared to be favorably impressed and subsequently suggested the possibility of using Indoklon by intravenous injection rather than inhalation. In his opinion, this method would be more acceptable to the psychiatrist than the inhalation technic.

We pursued this suggestion with vigor, realizing the difficulty involved in the injection of an insoluble ether like Indoklon into the blood stream. Many solvents were employed unsuccessfully. Ultimately, it appeared that polyethylene glycol 300 (Carbowax 300) was admirably suited for this purpose. This solvent is missible in all proportions with Indoklon. However, the most satisfactory solution for intravenous injection was found to be Indoklon 10%, Carbowax 300 56%, alcohol 10% and water sufficient to make 100%.

We established that when Indoklon is inhaled it is eliminated in the exhaled air. In order to ascertain the avenue of excretion when injected intravenously, a small cellophane bag containing a mouse was placed over the face of a dog, prior to the injection of Indoklon solution. At the moment the dog convulsed, the mouse likewise exhibited marked seizures from the inhalation of the exhaled Indoklon by the dog. This was repeated several times, indicating that intravenously injected Indoklon is excreted by the lungs in the exhaled air, as inhaled Indoklon is. Shortly thereafter the solution of Indoklon took its place alongside Indoklon, intended for inhalation, in the treatment of the mentally ill patients.

Having succeeded in giving an insoluble ether like Indoklon intravenously, we considered that certain ethers could be administered intravenously as anesthetics for surgical procedures. Such a method would present the advantages of simplicity of technic and accuracy of dosage measurement. We were unable to find a suitable solvent for the anesthetic ethers. Therefore, we attempted to emulsify a suitable anesthetic ether for intravenous injection. For our purpose, methoxyflurane appeared to be the most suitable agent.

The preparation of a suitable emulsion was difficult. It was necessary to add a vegetable oil to prevent hemolysis induced by the injected anesthetic. Ultimately, an emulsion containing 3.5% of methoxyflurane, 3% corn oil, with lecithin as the emulsifying agent, was selected as the most suitable formula. More than 150 dogs and several monkeys and rabbits were anesthetized with this anesthetic emulsion. Induction was rapid, anesthesia was smooth, and emergence was uneventful.[7]

In 1961, Dr. Helmut F. Cascorbi, who had worked with our group on this project, submitted himself as a volunteer to be anesthetized with this emulsion. With the cooperation of Dr. Martin Helrich, of the University of Maryland, the first anesthetic emulsion was administered to man successfully. This was followed with approximately 75 additional anesthesias. These were successful except for the production of embolic phenomena in a few individuals. At this time, the new amendment to the Food and Drug Act was passed, and the company supporting the project decided the risks were too great and withdrew its support. I have never concurred in this decision and feel that the problem of vein irritation and/or embolism production can be solved by additional research on the composition of the emulsion.

The advantages to be achieved by an acceptable solution to this problem are as follows:

1/ The use of high boiling point compounds as anesthetics that are unavailable by the inhalation technic.
2/ Flammability hazard is eliminated and the anesthetic "machine" is obviated.
3/ It is apparent that for surgical procedures in conditions of mass emergencies this procedure provides the advantage of simplicity with a minimum of equipment.
4/ For surgical procedures about the nose and mouth, this procedure permits the administration of a volatile anesthetic without the use of the anesthetic mask.
5/ A minimal amount of anesthetic is required, since when anesthesia is achieved the patient can be continued in the anesthetic state by allowing him to rebreathe the exhaled anesthetic.

It is my hope that someone will pursue this problem and bring it to a successful and practical solution.

Thus, in our studies of the fluorinated ethers and hydrocarbons, we took a roundtrip journey from anesthesia with Fluoromar and other fluorinated agents that eliminated the fire hazard from anesthesia. From there, via the fluorinated ethers, Indoklon was discovered as a new treatment in psychiatry for the mentally ill patient. And from psychiatry, having succeeded in developing an Indoklon solution available for intravenous use, our trip returned us to anesthesia, to the use of the volatile anesthetics given intravenously as emulsions. One is reminded of the timeless comment of the late Sir Frederick G. Hopkins, a distinguished English biological chemist, that is so fittingly applicable to the progress in pharmacology and anesthesiology:

> In a country rich in gold, an observant wayfarer may find a nugget here or there, but only the systematic mining will provide the currency of nations.

REFERENCES

1. Krantz, J. C., Jr., and Rudo, F. G.: The fluorinated anesthetics, *in* Eichler, O., ed.: Handbuch der Experimentellen Pharmakologie, vol. XX, chap. 10, Berlin, Springer, 1966, p. 502.

2. Robbins, B. H.: Preliminary studies of the anesthetic activity of fluorinated hydrocarbons, J Pharmacol Exp Ther *86:*197, 1946.

3. Krantz, J. C., Jr., Carr, C. J., Lu, G. G., and Bell, F. K.: Anesthesia XL, the anesthetic action of trifluoroethyl vinyl ether, J Pharmacol Exp Ther *108:* 488, 1953.

4. Krantz, J. C., Jr., Truitt, E. B., Jr., Speers, L., and Ling, A. S. E.: A new pharmacoconvulsive agent, Science *126:*353, 1957.

5. Krantz, J. C., Jr., Rudo, Frieda G., and Loecher, Claire K.: Anesthesia LXXI. Pharmacologic and psysiocochemical comparison of flurothyl and its isomer, Proc Soc Exp Biol Med *124:*820, 1967.

6. Ling, A. S. C., and Krantz, J. C., Jr.: The effect of bis (2-2-2-trifluroethyl) vinyl ether on brain electrolytes and water distribution in the rat, Biochem Pharmacol *12:*394, 1963.

7. Krantz, J. C., Jr., *et al.:* The intravenous administration of methoxyflurane emulsions in animals and man, Anesth Analg *41:*257, 1962.

CHAPTER

9

Anxiety and the Discovery of the Tranquilizers

F. M. BERGER, MD *

Human bondage consists in the impotence of man to govern or restrain the affects . . . for a man who is under their control is not his own master. A free man is one who lives according to the dictates of reason alone.
SPINOZA, 1670

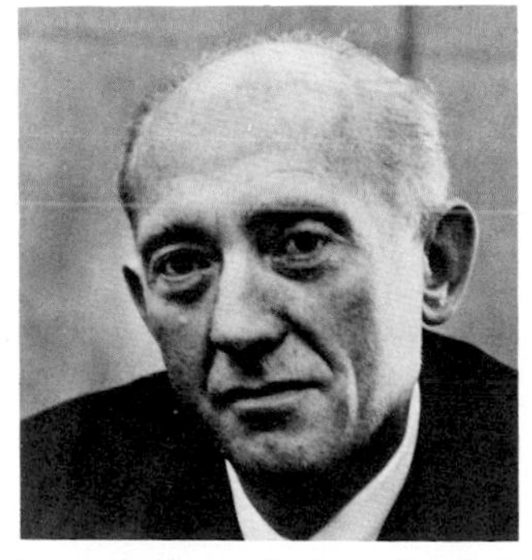

IF ANYTHING DISTINGUISHES MAN from animals, it is that humans are anxious. Animals react only to real dangers, or threats of it, by showing fear. Humans also react to unreal danger, or anticipation of it, by showing anxiety. Despite its wide prevalence, we do not generally understand the nature and meaning of anxiety. Several factors may account for this: our imperfect knowledge of the physiological and biochemical substrates of anxiety, the feeling that it may be primarily due to environmental factors, and the belief that anxiety, at least under some circumstances, may be a desirable and positive influence in life. Until recently it did not seem possible to do anything to specifically relieve anxiety. Drugs to treat this condition became available only during the last fifteen years. Since then they have been widely used. I would like to tell how this came about, describe how meprobamate, the first of

* President and Director of Research, Wallace Laboratories, Cranbury, New Jersey.

the antianxiety tranquilizers was discovered, and comment on the significance of this development.

ANXIETY, FEAR AND STRESS

Although the concept of anxiety has aroused psychiatric interest for more than 70 years, the term has been and is still used ambiguously (Lewis 1967). Different authors ascribe different meanings to it and often use the word interchangeably with the terms "fear" or "stress." Anxiety can be defined as an unpleasant feeling of apprehension, dread, or impending danger, which occurs in the presence of a recognizable threat. It may also occur in the absence of a threat or one that is, by reasonable standards, quite out of proportion to the emotion it evokes. Subjective bodily discomforts–such as a sense of constriction in the chest, difficulty in breathing or weakness in the legs–may also be present. Bodily disturbances, such as dryness of the mouth, sweating, tremor, palpitations, and other symptoms indicative of a dysfunction of the autonomic nervous system, may also occur but are not characteristic of anxiety as they may also be present in other emotional states (Altschule 1953). Fear, on the other hand, is an emotional response to a clearly recognizable and definite danger that threatens the individual.

It may not always be easy to differentiate fear from anxiety (Grinker and Spiegel 1945). In most instances, however, the distinction can be made. In anxiety, the organism reacts to a trivial danger as if it were a matter of life and death. Moreover, anxiety tends to be chronic and leads to inappropriate behavior, while fear is transient and preparatory to appropriate behavior. Stress, in the medical sense of the word, is the sum total of various bodily responses to stimuli that tend to alter the existing equilibrium. These stimuli need not be unpleasant.

THE PSYCHOANALYST'S CONCEPT OF ANXIETY

Freud considered anxiety as the fundamental, central problem of the psychoneurotic state. For many years he was preoccupied with its etiology. At first, he was convinced that it was due to tensions accumulated by frustrated sexual desires. Later he abandoned the concept of anxiety as transformed libido, and defined anxiety as a reaction to situations of danger. He distinguished between "neurotic" anxiety and fear, which he termed "realistic" or "objective" anxiety. He described realistic anxiety (fear) as a state due to actual known danger threatening from an external object. Neurotic anxiety, he now held, was anxiety about an unknown danger, something indefinite that lacks an object. It is a painful emotion evoked by one's own impulses that are perceived as the source of danger. By bringing this danger that is unknown to the patient into his consciousness, the analyst transforms neurotic anxiety into realistic anxiety. Elsewhere Freud expressed the idea that anxiety is the original reaction to helplessness that is subsequently reproduced in the danger situation as a signal for help.

While Freud and Ernest Jones on the whole made a distinction between fear, a normal phenomenon, and anxiety, which they considered morbid, many subsequent psychoanalytical writers did not do so. Others suggested that its origins were broader and that it was due to real or imagined disturbances in interpersonal relationships as well as inner conflicts. None of these ideas can be evaluated by direct experiments, so that it is difficult to assess their merit. If anxiety is indeed caused by repressed subconscious conflicts, a feeling of helplessness or by a disturbance of interpersonal relationships, it is difficult to see how tranquilizers would be useful in treatment. While these psychoanalytic interpretations may increase our understanding of the normal and diseased mental processes, they do not explain why some persons remain normal while others, under similar environmental conditions, become anxious and sick. Indeed, psychoanalysis and related therapies have been ineffective in the treatment of anxiety neurosis (Eysenck 1952).

ANXIETY AND MOTIVATION

In 1689, the English philosopher, John Locke, suggested that anxiety was the prime motive for human behavior. This belief persists today: it is still widely believed that anxiety is inherent in the solution of problems and that it sustains the creative drive, without which men would never survive (Rose 1958). If this were true and anxiety were such an important motivational force, it would be inappropriate to use drugs to affect it.

The role of anxiety as a motivational force is derived from Mowrer's (1939) reinterpretation of Freud's concept of anxiety in terms of a conditioned response. Miller *et al.* (1951) considered anxiety an acquired drive, which may be broadly defined as an anticipatory response to punishment, something that is essentially painful. Anxiety, therefore, is an anticipation of pain. According to this view, the visceral responses that sometimes accompany anxiety are characteristic of it and constitute innate or unlearned reaction to pain. The anxiety response is learned by associating other stimuli, such as fatigue, cold, hunger, and other unpleasant experiences, with pain itself. Anxiety thus becomes a conditioned response to symbols representing painful experiences.

This school of thought views anxiety as a drive that motivates behavior. Because anxiety represents a painful condition, its reduction is rewarding. Consequently, the individual learns to avoid anxiety by withdrawing from situations that are causing it. Thus, the function of anxiety is to serve as a signal for avoiding a situation of danger. Neurotic symptoms are created to remove or to rescue the ego from the situation of danger. Furthermore, anxiety is claimed to be responsible for the inhibition of sexual and aggressive impulses.

This whole argument rests on the assumption that anxiety is a conditioned fear-avoidance response that motivates behavior. The behavior therapy of psychiatric disorders has been developed on the basis of these theories. The specific methods of treatment utilized in psychoneurotic patients are desensitization and aversion therapy. In certain cases of phobia, where the obsessive fear is directed to a specific object or situation such as heights, open spaces or animals, these techniques have been effective. Behavior therapy has been of no value in the treatment of true anxiety states.

THE DEFINITION AND MEASUREMENT OF ANXIETY

Much of the disagreement among scientists about the meaning and nature of anxiety is due to the fact that many of the theories that have been offered cannot be tested by experiment. Anxiety cannot be precisely defined as long as we do not have reliable and verifiable data telling us something about the structure of this state. It is important to know whether there are one, two or many different kinds of anxieties, whether anxiety occurs only in normal or only in sick people or in both, and whether it is a normal personality attribute or a disease or only a symptom of a disease.

Reliable answers to these questions have been obtained by the employment of a statistical method called factor analysis. Factor analysis measures specific manifestations in a field and finds out which of these go together. It recognizes that any concept must represent, in the first place, a functional unity and that there are reliable mathematical methods that will indicate which attributes belong together. This multivariate experimental method does not start with guesses or postulates regarding particular concepts, but demonstrates by analysis of covariance what functional unities exist and what attributes are associated with it. This is the method that was used in the development of the intelligence tests by demonstrating the existence of certain definite structures of human abilities. Utilizing this method, Cattell and his associates evaluated many specific manifestations of anxiety obtained from questionnaires, interviews and extensive, objectively measurable psychological, physiological and behavioral tests.

Utilizing this approach, Cattell and Scheier (1958, 1961) found that there is a single general reaction pattern representing the manifestations of anxiety and therefore deserving the name anxiety. Anxiety does not include, however, all the behavioral responses that some persons have called anxiety, such as stress, neuroticism or motivational strength. Some of the more important characteristics of anxiety are the following: a lack of confidence, a sense of guilt and worthlessness, an unwillingness to venture, a dependency, readiness to become fatigued, irritable and discouraged, uncertainty about one's self, suspicion of others and a general tenseness. Indeed, this sad picture describes anxiety as something very different from anxiety as a positive motivational force. Cattell's finding that there is only one kind of anxiety is very significant. When measured and analyzed in a large number of persons of various backgrounds and suffering from a variety of different diseases, anxiety is qualitatively the same and indistinguishable in its characteristics and nature from person to person. There is no factual evidence to support the idea that there are different kinds of anxiety such as neurotic anxiety, psychotic anxiety or necessary anxiety.

The Cattell studies answered the important question, "Is anxiety normal or is it a disease or a symptom of a disease?" by showing it to be a symptom of a disease. Anxiety is not present at all, or is only transiently and to a small extent, in normal healthy individuals. When it is present, it is usually one of the symptoms of a disease, such as neurosis, depression, or schizophrenia.

The third important finding of the Cattell study was the observation that anxiety was not a motivating force or a stimulus to achievement as has been suggested by some psychologists. Anxiety is not a specific drive, like sex, self-assertion, fear, or curiosity. It is the opposite of a motivational drive. The more creative men are less anxious than the less creative men (Berelson and Steiner 1964). Anxiety has a disruptive influence on the mind. Motivation organizes and initiates behavior; anxiety either disorganizes or is a symptom of disorganization.

THE BIOLOGICAL BASIS OF ANXIETY

It would be difficult to understand or to justify the use of drugs in anxiety states without assuming that this symptom, like other symptoms of diseases, is due to a biological disorder of the organism. Electrophysiological research indicates that anxiety is associated with increased reactivity of specific areas of the brain. Anxiety has been produced by electrical stimulation of certain nuclei of the thalamus and of the limbic structures. Repeated stimulation of a particular nucleus evokes precisely the same symptoms and their intensity is directly proportional to the strength of the electrical current applied (Delgado 1969). This indicates that there is a biological foundation underlying this state. In spontaneous anxiety these areas may be hyperexcitable to normal stimuli or may be activated by sensory inputs of greater than ordinary magnitude that are the result of symbolic evaluation of environmental happenings or situations.

Grey Walter has found that anxiety in humans can be permanently relieved with electrocoagulation of discrete areas made through electrodes implanted in the frontal lobes. Destruction of discrete parts of the thalamus produces relief from anxiety neurosis probably as a result of the interruption of tonic pathways to the frontal lobes (Delgado 1969).

Meprobamate has a selective action on those specific areas of the brain that represent the biological substrate of anxiety. It has a synchronizing effect on the spontaneous electrical potentials of the thalamus (Hendley *et al.* 1957), and this action appears present in those areas of the thalamus that have been shown by electrical stimulation to induce anxiety experimentally. Meprobamate also normalizes the reflex hyperexcitability of the hippocampus and of the limbic system (Kletzkin and Berger 1959), and in this manner directly affects those structures of the brain that on stimulation by electric current induce anxiety in humans and in apes. In addition, meprobamate depresses conduction in hyperexcitable or hyperirritable interneuronal circuits (Berger 1954) and in this manner perhaps interrupts the reverberation so characteristic of psychoneurotic disease. Thus, considerable evidence shows that anxiety is due to a dysfunction of a part of the brain and that it is a symptom of a disease state. Consequently, it should lend itself to medicinal treatment like many other symptoms of diseases.

MEPHENESIN AND MEPROBAMATE

I will now briefly tell how I recall the development of meprobamate. To do this I have to start with mephenesin because the synthesis and development of meprobamate was the result of a determined and systematic effort to produce a compound superior to mephenesin. Almost eleven years elapsed between the discovery of mephenesin and the day meprobamate was made available to physicians as a prescription drug in April, 1955.

Discoveries in medicine are often made in an indirect, roundabout way. Back in 1945 I did not have any plans to discover either a muscle relaxant or a tranquilizer. I was working as a pharmacologist at the British Drug Houses Ltd in London, where I collaborated with William Bradley, the Chief Chemist, on the development of new synthetic antibacterial agents. Penicillin had just been made generally available, and I participated in these efforts by showing that greatly increased yields of penicillin could be obtained by extracting it from solutions adjusted in acidity to minimize its instability (Berger 1944, 1945). Bradley felt that it should be possible to synthesize a compound that would affect the gram-negative bacteria not killed by penicillin. At that time, there was a disinfectant on the market in Great Britain that was advertised as being particularly effective in killing gram-negative rods unaffected by penicillin. The name of this product was Phenoxetol, and chemically it was a phenylglycol ether. Bradley felt that lengthening the carbon chain to give phenylglycerol ethers might produce compounds with superior antibacterial effects. This expectation was fulfilled to some slight extent (Hartley 1947). I thought it worth while to determine the toxicity of these compounds and to find out how they affected mice. The compounds, much to my surprise, produced reversible flaccid paralysis of the voluntary skeletal muscles unlike that I had ever seen before. I decided to study this phenomenon in greater detail and to find out how it was brought about.

Administration of these compounds in appropriate dosage by the oral or parenteral route to mice, rats or other small laboratory animals caused muscular relaxation and paralysis of all voluntary skeletal muscles. The animals lost their righting reflex so that they were unable to turn over when put on their back. Their muscles were limp and completely relaxed. Yet the animals appeared conscious. Their eyes were open and they appeared to follow what was happening around them. The corneal reflex was present and they were able to respond with some movement to painful stimuli. During paralysis, spontaneous respiration, although largely abdominal, was preserved. The heart beat was regular and there were no signs suggesting an involvement of the autonomic nervous system. After paralysis was present for minutes or hours—depending on the dose of drug given—there was spontaneous and complete recovery to the state the animal was in prior to administration of the drug.

The animals treated with mephenesin, the most thoroughly studied phenylglycerol ether, looked different from those given an hypnotic or anesthetic drug. First, there was no evidence of excitement after administration of mephenesin and other glycerol ethers like that observed after administration of barbiturates or other hypnotics or anesthetic substances. Second, these compounds had a quieting effect on the demeanor of the animals. This was also clearly noticeable after administration of small doses that did not produce paralysis or muscular impairment. This effect was described as tranquilization and it was mentioned as such in the first publication reporting the pharmacological effects of glycerol ethers (Berger and Bradley 1946).

I was unaware at this time that the paralyzing action of 3-phenoxy-1,2-propanediol, a compound closely related to mephenesin, was described 35 years earlier by Gilbert and Descomps (1910) in France. These authors administered the compound to guinea pigs and observed transient paralysis of limbs and loss of reflexes in these animals. They also noted anesthesia and complete immobility in rabbits and a hypothermic effect in dogs.

Mephenesin was introduced into clinical practice as an agent to produce muscular relaxation during light anesthesia (Mallinson 1947). Subsequently, it was found to produce interesting effects in a variety of neurological and psychiatric conditions by Berger and Schwartz (1948) and Gammon and Churchill (1949). It was of particular interest when it was shown that mephenesin could allay anxiety without clouding consciousness (Hay 1949; Schlan and Unna 1949) and that it could induce in tense and anxious patients the state of relaxation characteristic of normal, healthy human beings (Dixon *et al.* 1950).

Yet, the drug had at least three drawbacks. It had a very short duration of action, it affected the spinal cord more than supraspinal structures, and it was not very potent so that large doses were required. To overcome these disadvantages, an extensive program of research was started with two goals in mind. The first one was the elucidation of the rapid breakdown of mephenesin in the body. It was felt that a more detailed knowledge of the metabolic fate of mephenesin would lead to the preparation of similar compounds with a longer duration of action since these new substances would not be degraded along the same metabolic pathways. The second approach was to evaluate a number of related compounds in the hope of finding one that would have a stronger muscle relaxant action and also exercise a stronger interneuronal blocking action on supraspinal structures.

Mephenesin proved to be one of the most rapidly absorbed drugs. A metabolic breakdown product of mephenesin was present in the urine of human subjects as early as 15 minutes after oral ingestion of the drug (Berger and Schwartz 1948; Berger 1949a) (Fig. 1). These compounds were identified as β-o-toloxylactic acid (Graves *et al.* 1948; Riley and Berger 1949) and β-(p-hydroxy-o-methyl-phenoxy) lactic acid (Riley 1950a and 1950b). Neither of these metabolites possessed mephenesin-like activity in the mouse.

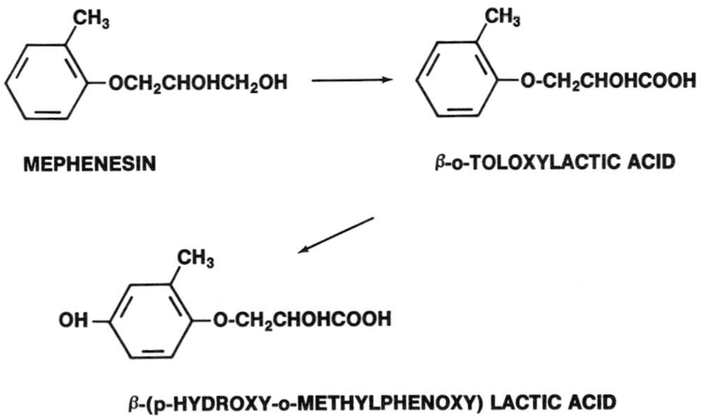

CH_3 –$OCH_2CHOHCH_2OH$ → CH_3 –$O\text{-}CH_2CHOHCOOH$

MEPHENESIN β-o-TOLOXYLACTIC ACID

CH_3 OH– –$O\text{-}CH_2CHOHCOOH$

β-(p-HYDROXY-o-METHYLPHENOXY) LACTIC ACID

Fig. 1. The metabolism of mephenesin.

Thus, the short duration of action of mephenesin was due to the rapid oxidation of the primary hydroxyl group to the lactic acid derivative.

It was considered worth while to attempt the preparation of longer-acting drugs of this type by making the terminal hydroxyl group less accessible to metabolic attack by esterifying it with a suitable acid. Various compounds of this type were prepared and studied. The acid succinate of mephenesin, as predicted, showed a significantly longer duration of action than the parent compound but its paralyzing action was even weaker than that of mephenesin itself (Berger and Riley 1949) (Fig. 2). The carbamate esters of

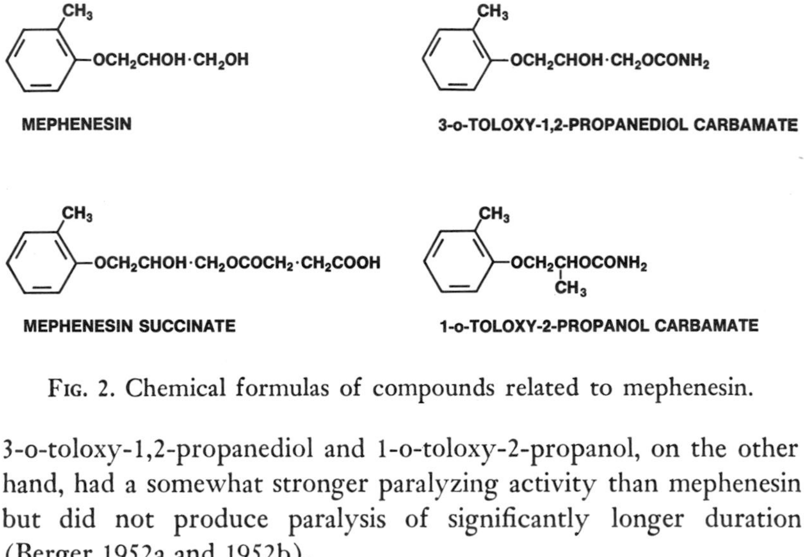

CH_3 — $OCH_2CHOH{\cdot}CH_2OH$

MEPHENESIN

CH_3 — $OCH_2CHOH{\cdot}CH_2OCONH_2$

3-o-TOLOXY-1,2-PROPANEDIOL CARBAMATE

CH_3 — $OCH_2CHOH{\cdot}CH_2OCOCH_2{\cdot}CH_2COOH$

MEPHENESIN SUCCINATE

CH_3 — $OCH_2CHOCONH_2$ (CH_3)

1-o-TOLOXY-2-PROPANOL CARBAMATE

FIG. 2. Chemical formulas of compounds related to mephenesin.

3-o-toloxy-1,2-propanediol and 1-o-toloxy-2-propanol, on the other hand, had a somewhat stronger paralyzing activity than mephenesin but did not produce paralysis of significantly longer duration (Berger 1952a and 1952b).

The mode of action of mephenesin at that time was quite well understood. It was known to affect multineuronal spinal reflexes and reduce reflex hyperexcitability (Berger 1947), and it was understood that these effects were primarily due to a selective depressant action on interneuronal circuits (del Castillo 1948). Although elegant methods for measurement of these effects were available, it was decided to evaluate compounds primarily by their ability to produce reversible paralysis of voluntary muscles. A compound was considered to have a potential as a tranquilizer when it produced loss of the righting reflex in mice without causing significant excitement prior to the onset of paralysis. All compounds were also evaluated for their ability to counteract pentylenetetrazol convulsion, which was considered an index of supraspinal central nervous depressant action.

Most ethers of glycerol, trimethylene glycol, and propylene glycol produced transient paralysis qualitatively similar to that observed after mephenesin (Berger 1948; Lott 1948). The glycol, erythritol and mannitol homologues of mephenesin had a weaker paralyzing action than the parent compound. It also became apparent that activity could not be substantially increased by variation of the substituents of the C_1 atom (Berger 1948). Substitution on the C_2 carbon of 1,3-propanediol, however, yielded compounds with interesting muscle relaxant and anticonvulsant properties and a more potent action on supraspinal levels than on the spinal cord (Berger 1949b).

My close collaboration with Dr. B. J. Ludwig started at about this period, during the second half of 1949. He was responsible for the preparation of all compounds evaluated since then; he first synthesized meprobamate in May, 1950. His contribution, however, went far beyond that. He and I discussed every one of the many decisions that had to be made along the way. His counsel, his clarity of thought, and his overall contribution to the success of the project were all-important, and I have been very fortunate in having him as a collaborator.

By this time it became clear that the 2-substituted 1,3-propanediols were of little practical interest because of their very short duration of action. The rapid metabolism and short duration of action were due, as was the case with mephenesin, to the rapid oxidation of the terminal hydroxyl groups. The diacetate of 2,2-diethyl-1,3-propanediol appeared to have a more prolonged action than the parent compound (Berger and Ludwig 1950)) but clinically did not have a sufficiently strong antianxiety effect (Selling unpublished). Several dicarbamates of 2-substituted 1,3-propanediols were longer acting and had stronger anticonvulsant action than the corresponding diols (Berger 1952a). Of these, the 2-methyl-2-n-propyl-1,3-propanediol dicarbamate (Ludwig and Piech 1951) was best and was selected for further study. It soon became apparent that this compound, called "Miltown" at that time and subsequently given the generic name "meprobamate," possessed a muscle relaxant and sedative action of an unusual kind (Berger 1954) (Fig. 3). Meprobamate had a duration of action about eight times longer than mephenesin. Like the parent drug, it depressed multi-

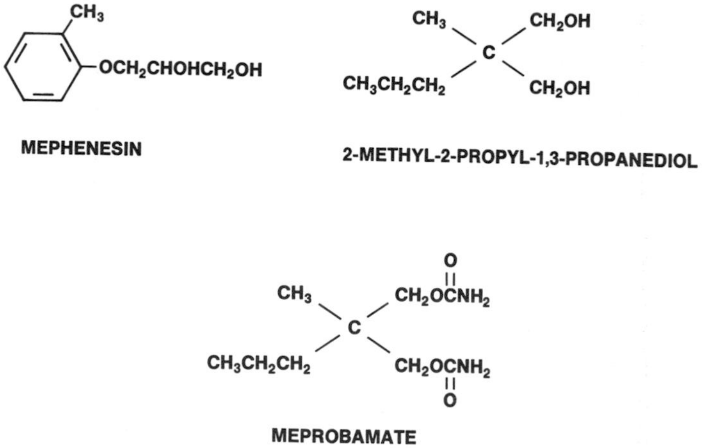

CH_3 —$OCH_2CHOHCH_2OH$

MEPHENESIN

CH_3, CH_2OH, C, $CH_3CH_2CH_2$, CH_2OH

2-METHYL-2-PROPYL-1,3-PROPANEDIOL

CH_3, CH_2OCNH_2 (=O), C, $CH_3CH_2CH_2$, CH_2OCNH_2 (=O)

MEPROBAMATE

FIG. 3. Chemical structure of mephenesin and meprobamate.

neuronal reflexes but did not significantly affect monosynaptic reflexes. It was readily and reliably absorbed from the gastrointestinal canal. It also had a taming effect. Monkeys after having been fed meprobamate lost their visciousness and could be more easily handled (Berger 1954). It had a selective action on the thalamus (Hendley *et al.* 1957) and on the limbic system of the brain (Kletzkin and Berger 1959).

SIGNIFICANCE OF TRANQUILIZERS

The discovery of antianxiety drugs is important from at least two points of view. First, tranquilizers like meprobamate specifically counteract anxiety. They are able to exert this effect without affecting other emotions, such as fear, without decreasing awareness of the environment and without impairing physical and intellectual performance (Berger and Potterfield 1969). In this respect, these drugs differ substantially from barbiturates, which have different properties and different uses (Berger 1963). Meprobamate, and perhaps the more recently developed antianxiety tranquilizers as well, have different uses from those of barbiturates because they act on different structures of the central nervous system (Berger 1968). Meprobamate has a selective action on those specific areas of the brain, such as the thalamus and limbic system, that represent the biological substrate of anxiety.

Second, the effects observed after administration of meprobamate are greatly influenced by the emotional stability of the subject.

Barbiturates and alcohol affect both emotionally stable and unstable individuals. Meprobamate, on the other hand, produces few if any noticeable subjective changes or objectively measurable behavioral effects in emotionally stable individuals. The drug improves performance, persistence, and behavior of emotionally unstable individuals so that they, under the influence of meprobamate, react like emotionally stable individuals (Marquis *et al.* 1957; Costello 1962b; Uhr *et al.* 1964; Janke 1960 and 1966). Emotionally stable subjects cannot feel the difference between meprobamate 400 mg and a placebo, while anxious subjects have no difficulty in distinguishing between them (Clyde 1960; Klerman *et al.* 1960; Hubin and Servais 1965).

Meprobamate neither interferes with nor facilitates performance of tasks done under threat of physical punishment (Pronko and Kenyon 1959). It is without significant effect in situations in which stress is induced by fatigue (Holliday and Devery 1962), physical pain (Knopf *et al.* 1959), social disapproval (Lienert and Thorgersen 1960), or unanticipated presentation of taboo words (Peterson *et al.* 1962). Thus, the unique and most significant feature of the action of meprobamate is its specificity: it is effective only in anxious patients and it affects only those areas of the brain that are involved in anxiety.

Koestler has aptly pointed out in "The Ghost in the Machine" that it would be wrong and naive to expect drugs to endow the mind with new insights, philosophic wisdom, or creative power. These things cannot be provided by pills or injections. Drugs can, however, eliminate obstructions and blockages that impede the proper use of the brain. Tranquilizers, by attenuating the disruptive influence of anxiety on the mind, open the way to a better and more coordinated use of the existing gifts. By doing this, they are adding to happiness, human achievement, and the dignity of man.

REFERENCES

1. Altschule, M. D.: Bodily Physiology in Mental and Emotional Disorders, New York, Grune, 1953.
2. Berelson, B., and Steiner, G. A.: Human Behavior–An Inventory of Scientific Findings, New York, Harcourt, 1964.
3. Berger, F. M.: Nature (London) *154:*459, 1944.
4. ——: Brit Med J *1:*116, 1945.
5. ——: Brit J Pharmacol *2:*241, 1947.
6. ——: J Pharmacol Exp Ther *93:*470, 1948.

7. ——: *Ibid. 96:*243, 1949a.
8. ——: Proc Soc Exp Biol Med *71:*270, 1949b.
9. ——: J Pharmacol Exp Ther *104:*229, 1952a.
10. ——: *Ibid. 104:*468, 1952b.
11. ——: *Ibid. 112:*413, 1954.
12. ——: Clin Pharmacol Ther *4:*209, 1963.
13. ——: *In* Efron, D. H., ed.: Psychopharmacology (A Review of Progress 1957-1967), Superintendent of Documents, Washington, DC, 1968, p. 139.
14. Berger, F. M., and Bradley, W.: Brit J Pharmacol *1:*265, 1946.
15. Berger, F. M., and Ludwig, B. J.: J Pharmacol Exp Ther *100:*27, 1950.
16. Berger, F. M., and Potterfield, J.: *In* Evans, W. O., and Kline, N. S., eds.: The Psychopharmacology of the Normal Human, Springfield (Ill), Thomas, 1969, p. 38.
17. Berger, F. M., and Riley, R. F.: J Pharmacol Exp Ther *96:*269, 1949.
18. Berger, F. M., and Schwartz, R. P.: JAMA *137:*772, 1948.
19. Cattell, R. B., and Scheier, I. H.: Psychol Rep (Monograph Suppl 5) *4:*351, 1958.
20. ——: The Meaning and Measurement of Neuroticism and Anxiety, New York, Ronald, 1961.
21. Clyde, D. J.: *In* Uhr, L., and Miller, J. G., eds.: Drugs and Behavior, New York, Wiley, 1960, p. 583.
22. Costello, C. G.: Canad Psychiat Ass J Suppl 7:S35, 1962.
23. del Castillo, J.: Arch Med Exp (Madrid) *11:*363, 1948.
24. Delgado, J. M. R.: Physical Control of the Mind–Toward a Psychocivilized Society, New York, Harper, 1969.
25. Dixon, H. H., Dickel, H. A., Coen, R. A., and Haugen, G. B.: Amer J Med Sci *220:*23, 1950.
26. Eysenck, H. J.: The Scientific Study of Personality, London, Routledge and Kegan Paul, 1952.
27. Freud, S.: An Outline of Psychoanalysis, New York, Norton, 1949.
28. Gammon, G. D., and Churchill, J. A.: Amer J Med Sci *217:*143, 1949.
29. Gilbert, A., and Descomps, P.: Compt Rend Soc Biol *69:*145, 1910.
30. Graves, E. L., Elliott, T. J., and Bradley, W.: Nature (London) *162:*257, 1948.
31. Grinker, R. R., and Spiegel, J. P.: Men Under Stress, Philadelphia, Blackston, 1945.
32. Hartley, F.: Quart J Pharm Pharmacol *20:*388, 1947.
33. Hay, J.: Canad Med Ass J *60:*224, 1949.
34. Hendley, C. D., Lynes, T. E., and Berger, F. M.: *In* Himwich, H. E., ed.: Tranquilizing Drugs, Publication No. 46, Amer Ass for the Advancement of Sci, Washington, DC, 1957, p. 35.
35. Holliday, A. R., and Devery, W. J.: Clin Pharmacol Ther *3:*5, 1962.
36. Hubin, P., and Servais, J.: Psychopharmacologia (Berlin) 7*:*235, 1965.
37. Janke, W.: Med Exp (Basel) *2:*217, 1960.
38. ——: Psychopharmacologia (Berlin) *8:*340, 1966.
39. Klerman, G. L., Di Mascio, A., Havens, L. L., and Snell, J. E.: Arch Gen Psychiat (Chicago) *3:*4, 1960.
40. Kletzkin, M., and Berger, F. M.: Proc Soc Exp Biol Med *100:*681, 1959.
41. Knopf, I. J., Worell, J., and Wolff, H. D.: Arch Gen Psychiat (Chicago) *1:*630, 1959.
42. Koestler, A.: The Ghost in the Machine, New York, Macmillan, 1968.
43. Lewis, A.: Israel Ann Psychiat *5:*105, 1967.
44. Lienert, G., and Thorgersen, H.: Med Exp (Basel) *2:*77, 1960.
45. Locke, J.: *In* Hutchins, R. M., ed.: Great Books of the Western World, vol. 35, Chicago, Encyclopedia Britannica, Inc., 1952.
46. Lott, W. A.: Trans NY Acad Sci *11:*2, 1948.

47. Ludwig, B. J., and Piech, E. C.: J Amer Chem Soc *73*:5779, 1951.
48. Mallinson, F. B.: Lancet *1*:98, 1947.
49. Marquis, D. G., *et al.:* Ann NY Acad Sci *67*:701, 1957.
50. May, P. R.: Meaning of Anxiety, New York, Ronald, 1950.
51. Miller, N. E.: *In* Stevens, S. S., ed.: Handbook of Experimental Psychology, New York, Wiley, 1951, p. 435.
52. Mowrer, O. H.: Psychol Rev *46*:553, 1939.
53. Peterson, E. A., Haun, K., and Upton, M.: Psychopharmacologia (Berlin) *3*:173, 1962.
54. Pronko, N. H., and Kenyon, G. Y.: Psychol Rep *5*:217, 1959.
55. Riley, R. F.: J Amer Chem Soc *72*:5712, 1950a.
56. ——: J Pharmacol Exp Ther *99*:329, 1950b.
57. Riley, R. F., and Berger, F. M.: Arch Biochem *20*:169, 1949.
58. Rose, T. F.: Canad Med Ass J *78*:144, 1958.
59. Schlan, L. S., and Unna, K. R.: JAMA *140*:672, 1949.
60. Uhr, L., Platz, A., Fox, S. S., and Miller, J. G.: J Gen Psychol *70*:51, 1964.

CHAPTER

10

The Benzodiazepines

Irvin M. Cohen, MD *

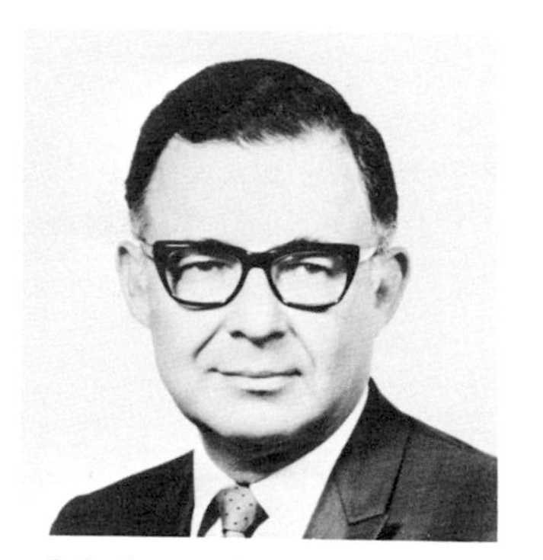

The prologue of the program of this symposium describes the speakers as discoverers coming together to tell the stories of their landmark achievements in biological psychiatry. Since I cannot claim the distinction of having originated the benzodiazepines as either chemicals or therapeutic agents, it is with considerable regret and indeed envy that I must disclaim the accolade of being called a "discoverer." My credentials for being here to relate the story lie in having had the good fortune to be given a very early opportunity to subject the first of the benzodiazepines, chlordiazepoxide, to clinical trial, and thereby to share in the excitement of determining that it was an active, therapeutically effective drug. Historically, the benzodiazepines have never been widely identified with specific persons, though obviously along the way outstanding individuals researched, developed, and clinically investigated them. The reason for this lies in the fact that the benzodiazepine story is essentially a model of how a therapeutic agent is conceived and brought forth by an enterprising pharmaceutical manufacturer who simply seeks to find a drug superior to others already in the marketplace. Participants in such group efforts often lose their opportunity for individual fame and renown, but in this instance the compensating reward was a major development in psychopharmacology that none could have accomplished alone.

* Clinical Associate Professor of Psychiatry, Baylor College of Medicine, Houston, and University of Texas Medical Branch, Galveston.

HISTORY

Credit for the actual discovery of the benzodiazepines belongs to Dr. Leo H. Sternbach, Director of Medicinal Chemistry in the Chemical Research Department in the Nutley, New Jersey, facilities of Hoffmann-La Roche Inc. However, the story really begins in Poland in the mid-thirties when Dr. Sternbach was working as a postdoctoral research assistant at the University of Cracow. At that time he was involved in synthesizing certain benzophenones, in the process of which he synthesized several compounds known as heptoxdiazines. Compounds of this type had been discovered in 1891 and their structure defined in 1924 as a seven-membered ring. Whether they were biologically active was then of no interest, since his concern lay entirely in the theoretical aspects of their chemistry. About 20 years later, in early 1954, this time in Nutley, New Jersey, in the laboratories of Hoffmann-La Roche, he resumed his interest in them, now with the hope of finding new compounds possessing psychopharmacologic activity. The effort was inspired largely by the phenomenal success of earlier tranquilizers such as the phenothiazine derivatives and meprobamate. The reasoning that led to his selecting as the target for his search a class of unexplored compounds with which he had worked 20 years earlier offers an interesting insight into the methods of modern pharmaceutical research. In seeking new therapeutic agents, the medicinal chemist has a choice of several routes. He may synthesize compounds structurally similar to naturally occurring products; an example of this is the chemical relationship of the synthetic anticholinergics and atropine. He may devise a working biologic hypothesis and apply compounds to it, as when Ehrlich's theory that bacteriophilic dyes might exert antibacterial activity led to the synthesis of Prontosil and ultimately the sulfa drugs. He may modify existing drugs to arrive at compounds of increased utility, as, for example, the improved semisynthetic penicillins derived from penicillin G. Or he may screen various chemicals in an attempt to find pharmacologically active substances that might prove therapeutic, essentially the approach taken by Dr. Sternbach. Classes of compounds ideal for random screening have certain special characteristics: they must be readily accessible, easily synthesized with good yields, and offer the possibility of many analogs that may be transformed into derivatives of various types.[1] The heptoxdiazines of his earlier years seemed ideal for the purpose since a search of the literature revealed no new members had been synthesized in the 20-year interval and their biological activities remained unknown.

His plan was to introduce a basic substituent into the heptoxdiazines, since it is generally recognized that basic substituents often impart biological activity. In the process, he discovered that the designated structure of the compounds that had been called heptoxdiazines for thirty years was actually incorrect. That is, they were not heptoxdiazines (seven-membered ring compounds) at all but quinazoline 3-oxides (six-membered ring compounds). This change in concept of the structure led to forty new derivatives; however, all of them proved pharmacologically inert. At this point he decided to abandon the study because of the disappointing results as well as demands imposed by other, more urgent projects. Near the end of 1955, in the very last experiment of the series, he decided to treat one of the quinazoline derivatives with a primary amine, methylamine, as against the previous use of various secondary and tertiary amines, which had produced such consistently negative results. The resulting compound, labeled Ro 5-0690, was then placed on the shelf and attention turned to more pressing research matters.

A year and a half later, in May, 1957, literally during a clean-up of the laboratory, Dr. Sternbach's chemist suggested that Ro 5-0690 be submitted for pharmacologic evaluation inasmuch as the chemical analysis was already complete. Identified only as "a white crystalline powder water soluble as the hydrochloride," it was sent on to the laboratory of Dr. Lowell O. Randall, Roche's Director of Pharmacologic Research. Two months later, on July 26, 1957, Dr. Randall wrote words now considered historic in the benzodiazepine story: "The substance has hypnotic, sedative, and antistrychnine effects in mice similar to meprobamate. In cats it is about twice as potent in causing muscle relaxation and ten times as potent in blocking the flexor reflex." As one might imagine, the unexpected finding of a pharmacologically active compound after a heretofore fruitless search generated considerable interest and enthusiasm. Further chemical studies revealed that Ro 5-0690 did not have the molecular configuration of a quinazoline 3-oxide, unlike the 40 inert compounds that preceded it. On the contrary, it became clear that it was an entirely new compound, formed by an unexpected molec-

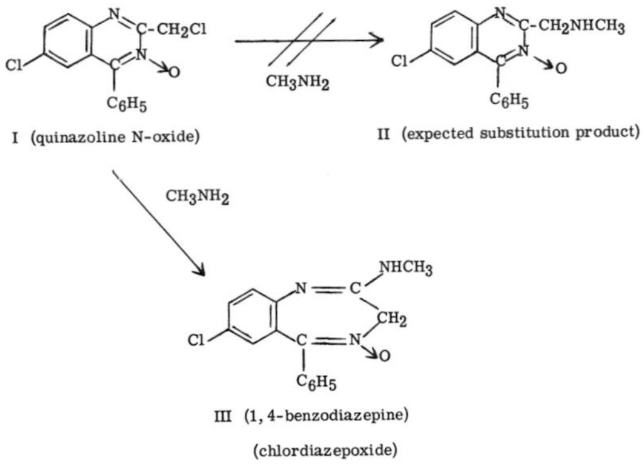

FIG. 1. Rearrangement of the quinazoline N-oxide.

ular rearrangement. By March, 1958, the structure was correctly identified as 1,4-benzodiazepine. Thus, its chemical structure was not definitely known until nearly a year after Dr. Randall uncovered its pharmacological activity. (Figure 1 shows the normal substitution product that was expected, and that which actually resulted, 1,4 benzodiazepine. Note that a novel ring enlargement had occurred, expanding from a 6- to a 7-membered ring.) With the urging of Dr. Randall and Dr. L. R. Hines, Director of Biologic Research, more detailed pharmacological and toxicity studies were undertaken.

The preclinical phase now completed, the clinical phase began. In early 1958, the drug was administered in fairly large doses to a few geriatric patients in two separate medical facilities. Early clinical results indicated the compound had marked sedative properties, but at the doses employed the patients also had severe ataxia and slurred speech. It was therefore discouragingly reported to be merely a simple sedative having no additional clinical interest. As a result of this pessimistic report nothing further was done for several months. This is perhaps a classic example of what may happen when the wrong dose is given the wrong type of patient. Dr. Hines was then placed in charge of further investigation of Ro 5-0690 plus two chemically unrelated compounds synthesized in the Basle, Switzerland laboratories of Hoffmann-La Roche. In general, the investigational plan was to give two of the compounds to a limited number of clinical investigators with the request that both compounds be tried simultaneously in patients in the diagnostic categories most frequently seen in the office practice of psychiatry, rather than in hospitalized mental patients. Dr. Hines offered two of the compounds to me for clinical trial, two to the late Dr. Titus H. Harris at the University of Texas Medical Branch in Galveston, and two to Dr. James R. Sussex, then at the University of Alabama School of Medicine in Birmingham. I had previously worked in Galveston with chlorpromazine and other phenothiazine derivatives and was satisfied that many good drugs were already available for the treatment of major mental disorders. I had also worked with meprobamate, a drug vastly superior to the barbiturates in treating the more frequently encountered psychiatric patient, the ambulatory psychoneurotic. However, a great need still existed for a drug having a midrange potency between meprobamate and the phenothiazines. Meprobamate was often too weak, the phenothiazines frequently too strong. Furthermore, the phenothiazines had too many side effects and potential complications to warrant regular use in the office patient. For this reason I was quite interested in investigating the new drugs that Dr. Hines believed might prove valuable in this indication. Very quickly it became apparent that Ro 5-0690, or methaminodiazepoxide as it was called for a short time, was an active compound. It was effective in controlling tension and anxiety, and did so with a minimum of side reaction. Its therapeutic spectrum exceeded that of meprobamate and approached that of the phenothiazines. Its therapeutic index (the ratio of therapeutic to toxic dose) was reasonably high. Most important, the calming action was accomplished in the same fashion as that of the tranquilizers: without clouding consciousness or interfering with intellectual acuity. The few side effects were almost totally dose related, and none of my patients experienced an adverse reaction. This added up to an easily manipulated drug having a wide latitude of clinical application and minimal toxicity. After a remarkably short period of exploration, each of the three investigators to whom the drugs had been given found chlordiazepoxide to have such interesting anxiolytic properties that work on the second compound given him was abandoned. Later, in a joint effort, Dr. John Kinross-Wright, Dr. James A. Knight, and I applied the drug independently in three settings: prison, clinic, and private office, and found our results consensually validated. Simultaneously, Dr. Harris in Galveston was sufficiently encouraged by his results to submit a clinical note to the *Journal of the American Medical Association.* It appeared in the March 12, 1960 issue, and was the first published announcement that the drug was therapeutically effective.[3]

Under the energetic direction of Dr. Hines, clinical trials were rapidly expanded so that by the end of 1959 sufficient experience had been assembled to permit a symposium on this new drug. In a memorable meeting held at the University of Texas Medical Branch in Galveston on November 13-15, 1959, chaired by Dr. Harris, a series of clinical reports was given on the antianxiety, muscle-relaxant, and anticonvulsant effects of the compound. Eventually, several thousand patients were treated in what now would be termed Phase III of the clinical investigation. On February 24, 1960, the New Drug Application was approved by the Food and Drug Administration, and a month later it was introduced as Librium. Its immediate acceptance by the medical profession revealed the unfulfilled need for an effective anxiety-reducing agent. It is now said to be one of the most widely prescribed drugs in the world, which is perhaps a commentary on our times.[4]

The pace of benzodiazepine research naturally quickened following the success of Librium. Fifty-five new benzodiazepine derivatives were synthesized. The first to show significantly greater activity than chlordiazepoxide was diazepam, which was synthesized by Dr. Sternbach in 1959. Despite the absence of many of the complicated structural features found in chlordiazepoxide, diazepam not only retained the tranquilizing property of chlordiazepoxide but in laboratory tests was five times more potent. It was also five times stronger as a muscle relaxant and ten times stronger as an anticonvulsant. Based on these findings it was expected to be a more potent tranquilizer clinically and possibly a useful muscle relaxant and anticonvulsant, predictions that were later confirmed clinically. In December, 1963, it was introduced as Valium.

The third benzodiazepine to become available in the US was oxazepam. It was synthesized in 1961 by Dr. S. C. Bell of Wyeth Laboratories. It resembles diazepam structurally but in clinical use its pharmacological activity is more comparable to chlordiazepoxide. It was placed in clinical trial in September, 1961, and reported at approximately the same time by Dr. Joseph Tobin and Dr. Sidney Merlis to be an active drug. In June, 1965, it was marketed as Serax.

In Europe, three other benzodiazepines are available. Nitrazepam, marketed by Roche as Mogadon, is a hypnotic. Medazepam, mar-

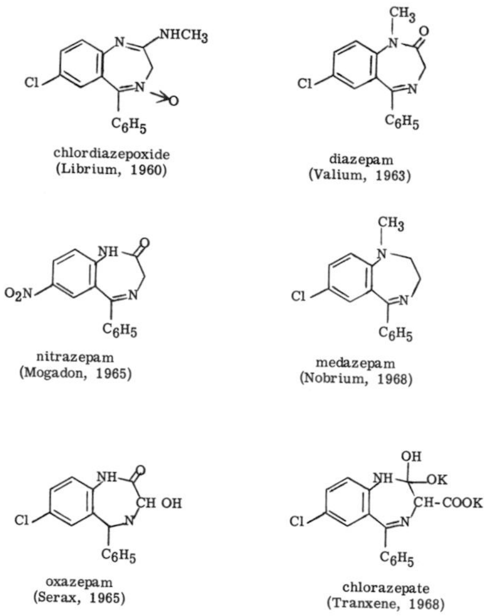

chlordiazepoxide
(Librium, 1960)

diazepam
(Valium, 1963)

nitrazepam
(Mogadon, 1965)

medazepam
(Nobrium, 1968)

oxazepam
(Serax, 1965)

chlorazepate
(Tranxene, 1968)

FIG. 2. Six benzodiazepines presently available.

keted as Nobrium also by Roche, is a tranquilizer similar in potency to Librium. Chlorazepate, a Librium-like compound, is marketed by a French pharmaceutical concern as Tranxene (see Fig. 2).

Thus, the early history of the benzodiazepines contains all the elements of drama that have characterized so many historical medical discoveries: exploration of the unknown, disillusionment and disappointment, abandonment of the project and rediscovery of a discarded compound, excitement in the laboratory followed by discouragement from the clinic, and eventual confirmation of the faith of early supporters. In the sixteen years since Dr. Sternbach resumed his work with a long ignored group of chemicals that was to yield an entirely new series of therapeutic agents, numerous benzodiazepines have been discovered. Hoffmann-La Roche alone has subjected over 1,500 to pharmacologic testing since 1957. Only about twenty have proved sufficiently interesting to be tested clinically. Research presently is directed toward developing analogs that show greater or lesser activity in each of the various parameters of their pharmacologic action. From this it is hoped that additional anxiolytics, hypnotics, anticonvulsants, muscle relaxants and perhaps even neuroleptics may be developed. The psychostimulant property that has been demonstrated in animals but that is less definite in humans, some say, may yet turn out an antidepressant agent.

PRESENT STATUS

In pursuit of the historical perspective of this symposium, it is appropriate to attempt to assess the present position of the benzodiazepines in therapeutics after a decade of usage. Four clinical applications of the benzodiazepines have stood the test of time: reduction of *1*/ anxiety and agitation, *2*/ the complications of acute alcoholism, *3*/ convulsive states, and *4*/ muscular tensions. Of these there is no doubt but that the outstanding property remains the capacity to reduce tension and anxiety. This so-called anxiolytic effect has been confirmed in numerous studies. Results are consistently reported to be most favorable in those states in which anxiety is free-floating, ego is well preserved, and the emotional disturbance is only partly disabling. Since these are precisely the same qualifications for positive results from, say, barbiturates, does it not follow that benzodiazepines are simply slightly improved sedatives and little more? If the term "sedative" is used in the context of being any drug that promotes relaxation by decreasing restlessness and irritability, then operationally the benzodiazepines are indeed simply sedatives. In fact, I find it convenient to teach that all psychotropic agents are merely better nonspecific sedatives then we have ever had, differing from one another only in their potency against anxiety, agitation, and aggression. If used in a more limited sense to imply that the older sedatives and the benzodiazepines are functionally interchangeable, then the term is no longer applicable. In everyday psychiatric practice, the therapeutic index of barbiturates, for example, is simply too low to deal adequately with the level of anxiety most patients present. Furthermore, the capacity of the cortical depressants to impair cognitive function and cloud consciousness, their higher potential for abuse, and potential lethality of overdoses relegate barbiturates and similar agents to the position of being almost anachronistic in managing the nonhospitalized patient. Of all the so-called antianxiety drugs available at this time, in my opinion the benzodiazepines offer the greatest latitude of application, predictability of action, and freedom from adverse effects in the management of neurotic anxiety.

All three of the currently available benzodiazepines possess anticonvulsant properties. However, only diazepam has found widespread use in the treatment of convulsive states. Its effectiveness in terminating status epilepticus has been amply documented and many consider it the drug of choice.[5,6] On the other hand, the value of the benzodiazepines as prophylactics in epilepsy is still in doubt. Early studies of differential effects of benzodiazepines on chemically and electrically induced seizures in animals led to predictions of specificity.[7] For example, the parallel effectiveness of trimethadione and the benzodiazepines against Metrazol-induced seizures suggested that they would be particularly useful against petit mal epilepsy. Predictions of this sort have been substantiated to some extent clinically, and various reports do show best results in protecting against myoclonic, petit mal, and psychomotor seizures.[8,9] However, the accumulated data has not yet been sufficiently impressive to establish superiority over drugs traditionally used in prophylactic regimens. The prevailing view is that in man benzodiazepines possess broad spectrum anticonvulsant properties and are best used as adjuncts rather than as the principal medication. This adjunctive role has led some to conclude that their actual anticonvulsant action is clinically negligible and what there is depends mainly on the psychosedative properties, that is, on the elimination of tension and anxiety that so often interferes with seizure control. Militating against this is the superiority of diazepam, the strongest available benzodiazepine, over diphenylhydantoin and phenobarbital in status epilepticus.[10] The question of why diazepam is better at stopping seizures than preventing them is also unsettled. Perhaps it relates to the relatively brief peak action, and a sustained-action preparation is needed. More likely the answer will come when a benzodiazepine analog having really potent and sustained anticonvulsant activity is developed.

The tranquilizers in general have proved of inestimable value in the treatment of acute disorders associated with alcoholism. Nothing in the management of withdrawal symptoms and various acute brain syndromes such as delirium tremens and acute hallucinosis has ever been as effective or safe. Kaim *et al.* recommend chlordiazepoxide as the drug of choice on the basis of a statistically significant reduction in withdrawal seizures and incidence of delirium tremens, plus the fact that risks associated with the use of chlorpromazine are avoided.[11] Other studies report that chlordiazepoxide and diazepam may lower relapse rate in chronic alcoholism. The validity of experimental findings in such a complex disease as alcoholism requires extended study. The value of chlordiazepoxide, oxazepam, and diazepam in the treatment of acute alcoholism and its complications is unquestionable, though there is no proof that they are superior to other psychotropic drugs, particularly chlorpromazine. Their use in chronic alcoholism remains as much an arguable issue as it is with any other psychotropic drug.

It is generally agreed that the ideal muscle relaxant is yet to be developed. The major defect in those presently available is unpredictability of degree and quality of response. The problem of developing a generally satisfactory relaxant is complicated by many factors, including poor correlation between animal test and clinical experience, the variety of physiological levels at which muscular disorders occur, the numerous etiologies, and the multiple associated factors such as pain, anxiety, nutritional status, general state of the patient's health, etc. Evaluating muscle-relaxant action is often imprecise due to difficulties in separating sedative and muscle-relaxant properties. At this time the benzodiazepines, particularly diazepam, are in wide use. There is abundant evidence demonstrating they are clinically effective in many neuromuscular conditions, including spasticity of serious degree such as may be found in tetanus and upper motor neuron paralyses.[12-14] Less severe myalgias of musculoskeletal origin, such as those associated with low-back strain and cervical spasm, are also responsive, though in these conditions tranquilizing action may be as important as muscle-relaxing action.[15] Results in the treatment of cerebral palsy have been variable, some positive results possibly being secondary to psychosedative effects.[16] Rogers reported the muscle-relaxing capacities of diazepam were not significantly greater than those of methocarbamol and attributed the generally better results from diazepam to the superiority of its calming action.[17] A deterrant to the use of the benzodiazepines in many cases is the occurrence of troublesome side effects of drowsiness and incoordination at the level that satisfactory muscle relaxation may appear. In declaring the present status of the benzodiazepines as muscle relaxants, the consensus appears to be that they are at least as good as any available for most indications, and probably better in most.

In summary, the benzodiazepines appear to occupy a substantial but not necessarily unassailable position in therapeutics. They are useful drugs, and probably the best all-around pharmacotherapeutic agents available today for the relief of anxiety in nonpsychotic, ambulatory patients. In convulsive states, diazepam seems to be the drug of choice in terminating status epilepticus. Chlordiazepoxide, oxazepam, and diazepam are useful adjunctively in controlling epilepsy but as a rule are not so reliable as traditional anticonvulsants. As muscle relaxants, the benzodiazepines, particularly diazepam, are as good or perhaps better than any available. In the treatment of acute complications of alcoholism, they can be very useful, though it is doubtful that they are superior to chlorpromazine.

EPILOGUE

The development of the benzodiazepines is a major landmark in modern psychochemotherapy. The usefulness of this class of compounds, particularly as medicinals in emotional illness, depends on a broad spectrum of unique pharmacologic qualities that all members of the group possess. Their discovery was not the result of serendipity, nor were they the fruits of planned efforts to synthesize compounds patterned on the structures of naturally occurring compounds. Ironically, in the development of chlordiazepoxide, the first of this new class, serendipity might be said to have worked in reverse, namely that at two points in its development the drug came near to being overlooked or scrapped. That the compound was saved from such a fate is due to *1/* the recognition by a chemist that its chemical structure was *not* that of a group of pharmacologically inert compounds; *2/* an alert pharmacologist who detected its crucial pharmacologic properties; *3/* an energetic researcher who persisted in reinvestigating it, despite its failure in its initial clinical trials; and *4/* clinicians who called attention to its specific antianxiety effect in humans. From these early efforts has emerged a chain of compounds that has greatly improved the physician's capacity to help the anxious patient. Perhaps of more lasting significance is the part they will continue to play in the struggle to gain an understanding of the biological basis for man's emotions.

REFERENCES

1. Sternbach, L. H., Randall, L. O., and Gustafson, S. R.: *In* Gordon, M., ed.: Psychopharmacological Agents, vol. 1, New York, Acad Press, 1964, p. 137.
2. Kinross-Wright, J., Cohen, I. M., and Knight, J. A.: Dis Nerv Syst *21*:23, 1960.
3. Harris, T. H.: JAMA *172*:1162, 1960.

4. Ban, T.: Psychopharmacology, Baltimore, Williams & Wilkins, 1969, p. 326.
5. Bailey, D. W., and Fenichel, G. M.: J Pediatrics *73*:923, 1968.
6. Gastaut, H., Naquet, R., Poire, R., and Tassinari, C. A.: Epilepsia (Amst) *6*:167, 1965.
7. Swinyard, E. A., and Castellion, A. W.: J Pharmacol Exp Ther *151*:369, 1966.
8. Cohen, N. H., *et al.:* Dis Nerv Syst *22* (Suppl 7):20, 1961.
9. Liske, E., and Forster, M. J.: New Drugs *3*:241, 1963.
10. Lombroso, C. T.: Neurology (Minneap) *16*:619, 1966.
11. Kaim, S. C., Klett, C. J., and Rothfield, B.: Amer J Psychiat *125*:1640, 1969.
12. Herrero, J.: *In* Principles of Tetanus, Proc Intl Conf on Tetanus, Bern (Switzerland), Hans Huber Company, July, 1966, p. 535.
13. Peirson, G. A., Fowlks, E. W., and King, P. S.: Amer J Phys Med *47*:143, 1968.
14. Masterson, J. H., and White, A. E.: Med Times *92*:1194, 1964.
15. Katz, R. A., Aldes, J. H., and Rector, M.: J Neuropsychiat *3*:S91, 1962.
16. Engle, H. A.: Develop Med Child Neurol *8*:661, 1966.
17. Rogers, E. J.: Western Med *4*:11, 1963.

CHAPTER

11

Biological Research in the Pharmaceutical Industry with Reserpine

Hugo J. Bein, MD *

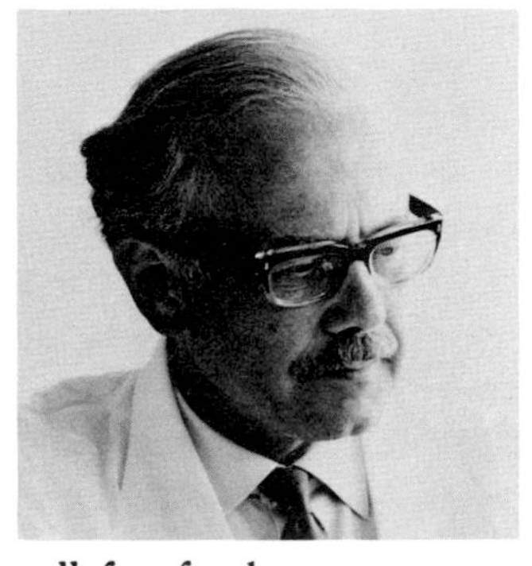

The invitation to this Symposium, which I deem it an honor to have received, was accompanied by the request that I give an account of the discovery of reserpine. I am afraid that a mere historical review would be of interest to no one—not even to the speaker—because the isolation of reserpine from the rauwolfia plant is a *fait accompli* that does not really call for further comment; a brief report on the alkaloid's isolation was published by Müller, Schlittler, and Bein in 1965.[9] Instead, I propose to discuss some of the lessons we at Ciba have learned in the course of our work on reserpine and to illustrate, by reference to the progress we have made in our department, what a decisive influence the knowledge that the world of science gained from reserpine has had on the discovery of new drugs.

"Primum et laudatissimum remedium" is the epithet applied to rauwolfia in a Portuguese work published in Goa as far back as 1563.[11] Although rauwolfia had repeatedly been described in books by herbalists down through the centuries, it was not until the 1940s that interest in this plant spread to scientific circles outside India.[1]

* The University of Basel Faculty of Medicine, Switzerland, Director of Biological Research, Ciba Ltd.

Indian research workers produced the first well-documented clinical findings. In India, rauwolfia was employed to sedate patients suffering from mental disorders, as well as to induce tranquilization; incidentally, it may be interesting to note that the term "tranquilizer" was coined in Ciba Summit in 1953 by F. F. Yonkman, in connection with the pharmacological characterization of reserpine. It was also an Indian author who first gave a detailed description of the antihypertensive action of reserpine, an action at that time that aroused particular interest in the West. Furthermore, many alkaloids have been isolated from the rauwolfia plant in India, but none has proved to be the therapeutically active substance. The aim of our team was to isolate the unknown active principle. This is identical with reserpine.[1] When reserpine was isolated, then, clinical confirmation of the two principal effects of rauwolfia had already been obtained.

After descriptions of reserpine had been published and the drug had become the object of widespread laboratory research and intensive clinical use, many institutes and institutions jumped to the conclusion that in the realm of so-called folk medicine or in medicine as practiced by primitive peoples there was probably an abundance of therapeutically valuable preparations of natural origin simply waiting, as it were, to be purified and investigated in the laboratory. A campaign was therefore duly launched with a view to combing through all possible types of plant, and expeditions were dispatched into regions in which little exploration had hitherto been undertaken. It is possible to gain only a fragmentary impression of the results yielded by this campaign, which set in throughout the world; from evidence of various kinds, however, it can be concluded that the effort expended must have been enormous, and that these attempts to discover new therapeutically active agents were not crowned with success.

For a number of years, we also participated in this international hunt. Finally, we realized what should in fact have been obvious to all concerned, namely, that the situation with regard to rauwolfia was fundamentally different as compared with all the other folk medicines or medicinal plants studied by us. In the case of rauwolfia, we had possessed, from the very beginning, evidence that—even considered by modern standards—could be taken as confirmation of its clinical activity. *Rauwolfia* was thus not simply a substance to be regarded as a candidate for "blind screening," but an agent calling for research along the lines of specific *ad hoc* analysis. This meant that we already had a proper basis for our pharmacological work; the difficulties encountered with the Rauwolfia plant lay in the fact that its principal active substance, reserpine, was relatively sparingly soluble and had a very gradual onset of effect, and that the Rauwolfia plant contained a wide variety of pharmacologically active compounds, some of which were found to antagonize certain of the effects of reserpine. Selecting the appropriate criteria of evaluation to be applied during the progressive purification of the active rauwolfia fractions was therefore of decisive importance.

It has always been my opinion that in the case of a centrally acting substance, the pattern of effects produced in the unanesthetized laboratory animal is of primary interest. For this purpose we worked largely with hare-rabbits, since this is a species with which it is possible to study, in one and the same animal, the effects exerted by a substance on a large number of functions—in much the same way as a clinician does with a patient. Among the functions we observed were: behavior, motor activity, muscle tone, reflexes (including light reflexes), body temperature, respiration, heart rate, etc. While studying total extracts of rauwolfia, we were struck by the fact that, though not suppressing normal ocular reflexes to light, they did cause pronounced contraction of the pupil—this usually being the first and most prolonged sign of their activity. When screening extracts for the purpose of concentrating the active component of rauwolfia, i.e. reserpine, we found that this miotic effect, together with the tranquilizing effect, provided us with our most important guiding clue.

The rauwolfia plant contains dozens of pharmacologically active substances; this genus of Apocynaceae is probably one of the most prolific single sources of alkaloids in the entire vegetable realm. Without entering into details, it can be said that, depending on the nature of the chemical processing employed, compounds of one or another type predominate, with the result that pharmacologically different patterns of effects are encountered. In the case of certain fractions, for example, the tranquilizing effect of the reserpine present in them was found to be masked by the action of central-stimulant substances. In the course of screening operations, we also observed extraordinarily inconsistent effects on the blood pressure: particularly marked interference was caused by substances displaying pressor activity, which are likewise present in rauwolfia. Even after reserpine had been successfully isolated in pure form, its typical hypotensive activity—owing chiefly to the slow onset of effect—could only be consistently reproduced provided meticulously controlled experimental conditions were adhered to. Screening of the various extracts for hypotensive activity alone would therefore have been unlikely to prove at all promising.

We conclude that the reason for the success of this pharmacological research lay in the fact that the extracts were not simply screened by reference to a particular effect, but that care was taken to make the pharmacological analysis of every preparation as comprehensive as possible, thereby enabling us to fit each of the individual effects into an overall picture and to determine their relative importance in each instance. Consequently, for the purposes of biological screening, we have since made it a practice to undertake the work of analysis on as broad a basis as possible, particularly when evaluating compounds purported to have a central action.

In terms of milligrams quantity, reserpine is a highly potent agent exhibiting both central and peripheral sites of attack. It initiated a new epoch in the treatment of arterial hypertension and, together with chlorpromazine, also in the treatment of psychiatric cases. Observations made in this country in 1955, namely, that reserpine causes a loss of 5-hydroxytryptamine from brain tissue,[10] as well as findings reported from Great Britain in 1956 [4] and, independently, from Sweden too,[3] that it also affects the concentration of noradrenaline in various tissues, marked the beginning of an entirely new era in our understanding of the physiology and pharmacology of the autonomic nervous system. Reserpine thus became an extremely important tool for the pharmacologist, a tool whose influence has been far reaching. It is difficult to imagine, for example, how our group in Ciba Summit could have discovered the potent antihypertensive agent guanethidine and analyzed its mechanism of action, if their research on reserpine had not already provided them with a basis upon which to work.

I should like to go beyond the confines of reserpine as a topic here and to devote a few remarks to a new therapeutically interesting category of substances that has been developed in our laboratories. That this new development was possible at all is thanks largely to the experience we had acquired with reserpine and to knowledge recently gained in the field of catecholamine metabolism, knowledge likewise ultimately attributable to research on reserpine.

Since the compounds that had to be evaluated were supposed to affect abnormal behavior in man, let us first review the situation in psychopharmacology. As realists, we have to acknowledge that one of the major difficulties encountered in this field is the fact that the etiology of aberrant behavior in man is still unknown; this, however, applies not only to pathological types of behavior, but also to numerous other diseases for which many effective drugs have nevertheless been developed. To complicate matters, the action of drugs on behavior is also still largely unexplored. This has led pharmacologists to characterize new drugs by reference to their similarity with other existing drugs, and various different avenues have accordingly been selected, depending on the personal preferences of the investigator concerned: some have chosen biochemical approaches and some have relied on behavioral techniques, either instrumental or observational, while others have based their research on the antagonistic effects exerted by the new substances on certain of the actions produced by well-known drugs, among which reserpine has generally been widely used.

In our primary screening procedures we have made use of possible antagonistic effects against stimulants or depressants as one of our main investigational pillars. In other words, we have to some extent been studying the behavior of new substances in animals rendered "abnormal" by other substances. This part of the screening schedule includes testing for an antagonistic effect against the stimulant action of mescaline on motor activity in mice. Here I am fascinated by the finding that psychopharmacological drugs that are alleged to be clinically active—whether as thymoleptics, like imipramine, or as neuroleptics, like reserpine—exert an antimescaline action in the mouse. The second pillar consists in meticulous observation of the pharmacological picture in experiments on nonanesthetized animals of the type to which I have already referred in connection with our testing of the various rauwolfia extracts.

Since our objective was to develop psychopharmacological agents differing from existing ones, we were especially interested in fundamentally new chemical structures, since it seemed likely that our requirements would best be fulfilled by new chemical entities. Our program with a novel chemical series of this kind started in 1960. One compound in this series—designated with our code number

27,937-Ba—looked especially attractive from an experimental point of view; it belongs to the new chemical class of the dibenzo-bicyclo-octadienes synthesized by Wilhelm and Schmidt.[12] An attempt has been made here to represent the chemical structure in a three-dimensional manner, so as to convey a more vivid idea of the molecule than possible by conventional means (Fig. 1). The basic chemical framework consists of several rings lying in different planes and arranged at particular angles to one another.

CIBA 27937 - Ba

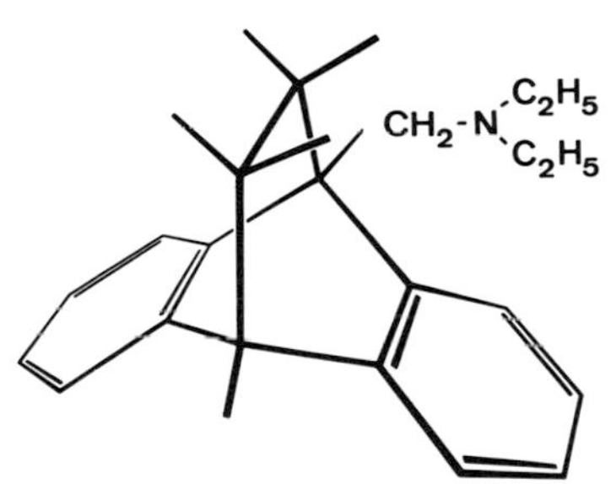

FIG. 1. Structural formula of CIBA 27,937-Ba, 1-diethyl-amino-methyl-dibenzo(b,e)bicyclo(2.2.2)octadiene.

27,937-Ba showed a peculiar type of central activity. It is neither a chlorpromazine-like nor an imipramine-like substance; in other words, it has its own distinctive pharmacological profile. All of us, chemists and biologists alike, eagerly awaited the feedback from clinical trials; I do not want to go into details and should only like to say that—although central effects, including some thymoleptic activity, were undoubtedly present in man—the substance did not prove of much therapeutic usefulness in these trials. Extrapolation from animal to man was thus unsuccessful with regard to the therapeutic value of this compound, but, at least in our eyes, the compound itself could be considered a success inasmuch as it appeared to provide a promising starting point for the synthesis of new analogs. The testing of these analogs revealed unsuspected and hitherto unknown relationships between chemical structure and pharmacological activity. I propose to illustrate this point by quoting the example of two closely related analogs of the first-mentioned compound. From the chemical standpoint, these two compounds differ in only one respect, namely, in their side chain,

CIBA 30803-Ba — TRANQUILIZER — CH_2-N(H)(CH_3)

CIBA 34276-Ba — THYMOLEPTIC — CH_2-CH_2-CH_2-N(H)(CH_3)

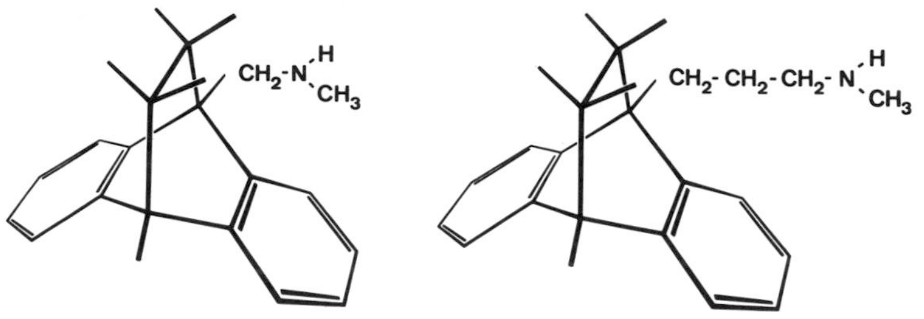

FIG. 2. Structural formula of CIBA 30,803-Ba, 1-methyl-amino-methyl-dibenzo(b,e)bicyclo(2.2.2)octadiene, and of CIBA 34,276-Ba, 1-methylaminopropyl-dibenzo(b,e)bicyclo(2.2.2)octadiene.

which in CIBA 34,276-Ba is extended by two CH_2 groups as compared with CIBA 30,803-Ba (Fig. 2). This chemical modification, though certainly only a minor one, induces marked qualitative changes. Before analyzing the pharmacological data, I should like to mention now that both substances are active in man and that, broadly speaking, compound 30,803-Ba can in a certain sense be classified as a tranquilizer [2] and compound 34,276-Ba as a thymoleptic.[5] This, however, does not imply that they behave exactly like substances that are already known. It would be beyond the scope of this lecture if I were to enumerate the ways in which these compounds also differ from established drugs.

The difference in the pharmacological picture of the two compounds becomes clearly evident when they are investigated in nonanesthetized animals, in neuropharmacological tests, in isolated organs, and in biochemical testing procedures. For the sake of simplicity, I do not propose to list all the tests that we carried out in this connection, but instead merely select a few typical ones.

In nonanesthetized animals, 30,803-Ba—i.e. the compound with the shorter side chain—produces muscle relaxation and tranquilization in a variety of species. Increasing the doses does not produce anesthesia. In contrast to 30,803-Ba, compound 34,276-Ba induces ataxia and hyperreflexia in low doses; higher doses of 34,276-Ba usually give rise to spasticity. No sedative action has been found with 34,276-Ba in any of the animal species studied. This very obvious qualitative difference between the two compounds, as revealed by gross observation, has also been encountered in a large number of neuropharmacological tests, such as:

tests on polysynaptic flexor reflex transmission in anesthetized cats or rabbits, and in decerebrate cats as well as high spinal cats;
tests on the tonic activity of individual gamma-motoneurones; and finally
tests on extensor rigidity in cats decerebrated by midbrain section and in cats decerebrated by anemia (Fig. 3).

Effect on :	CIBA 30803 - Ba	CIBA 34276 - Ba
Polysynaptic reflex transmission	Marked inhibition	Very slight occasional stimulation
Tonic activity of γ-motoneurones	Marked inhibition	Very slight
Decerebrate rigidity	Marked inhibition	Very slight

FIG. 3. Effect of CIBA 30,803-Ba and CIBA 34,276-Ba in various neuropharmacological test systems.

In all these tests, there is a marked difference between 30,803-Ba and 34,276-Ba:

30,803-Ba decreases polysynaptic reflex transmission in rabbits and cats. This reflex transmission is inhibited in the spinal cat to a much smaller extent than in the normal anesthetized cat—a fact that suggests that 30,803-Ba has a supraspinal site of attack.[2]
30,803-Ba also damps down the activity of tonically active gamma-motoneurones in cats decerebrated by midbrain section.[2]
In view of all these effects on motor control, it is not surprising that 30,803-Ba diminishes extensor rigidity in cats decerebrated by midbrain section or by anemia.

The pharmacological picture presented by 34,276-Ba in these same test systems is a radically different one:

Polysynaptic reflex transmission is inhibited by 34,276-Ba only in sublethal doses and, even then, only to a comparatively small extent; a stimulant action, at least in some experiments, is evident. 34,276-Ba exerts, at the most, only a very weak effect on decerebrate rigidity and on the gamma-fiber system.

There is nothing really so surprising about the fact that a relatively minor change in a given chemical structure may either enable certain pharmacological effects to emerge more strongly or, alternatively, cause them to disappear; many examples could be quoted to illustrate this type of phenomenon. But I can think of no example in which, as happens with our two compounds, a mere change in the structure of the molecule is sufficient to place the compound into a different therapeutic category within the CNS. This can be demonstrated experimentally by reference to the differing effects that the two compounds exert on catecholamine metabolism—which brings us back once again to reserpine and its repercussions on pharmacological research.

It can now be considered a well-accepted fact that psychopharmaceuticals have an influence on the adrenergic nervous system, including particularly an effect on the uptake, release, and turnover of catecholamines. This does not mean that a causal connection necessarily exists between their psychopharmacological activity and the influence they exert on the catecholamines, but simply that many centrally acting compounds are capable of affecting catecholamine metabolism.

CIBA 34,276-Ba, like imipramine, inhibits the uptake of noradrenaline in the rat heart; 30,803-Ba, on the other hand, in contrast to 34,276-Ba, is not active in this respect [7] (Fig. 4).

34,276-Ba also inhibits the uptake of noradrenaline in isolated granules from the sympathetic nerves of the bovine spleen. In this respect, 30,803-Ba is less active than 34,276-Ba.

The catecholamine content of the brain and of the heart is not significantly altered by single doses of 34,276-Ba and 30,803-Ba, even where high doses are given; only when repeated doses of 34,276-Ba are administered does some, but not very marked, de-

	CIBA 30803-Ba	CIBA 34276-Ba
I. Inhibition of noradrenaline (NA) uptake		
in situ	inactive	ACTIVE
isolated granules	slightly active	slightly active
II. Change of NA content of brain after repeated administration	inactive	slightly active (irregular)
III. Activation of tyrosine hydroxylase after single administration	ACTIVE	inactive

FIG. 4. Effect of CIBA 30,803-Ba and CIBA 34,276-Ba on the catecholamine metabolism in the rat.

crease occur in the noradrenaline content of the heart and of the brain; the dopamine content in the brain is not significantly reduced. 30,803-Ba has no demonstrable effect on the catecholamine content of the brain and heart.

Histochemical studies conducted on individual catecholamine-containing neurons have likewise revealed a clear-cut distinction between 30,803-Ba and 34,276-Ba. 34,276-Ba does inhibit the uptake of catecholamines by various noradrenaline neurons, whereas 30,803-Ba does not.[6]

When one probes deeper into an analysis of the action exerted by both drugs on catecholamine metabolism, a further distinction becomes evident insofar as 30,803-Ba interferes with catecholamine biosynthesis in the brain after pretreatment with single doses, whereas in this case it is 34,276-Ba that proves the inactive compound. 30,803-Ba activates tyrosine hydroxylase, an enzyme occupying the key position in the formation of catecholamines.[2,7]

Since single doses of 30,803-Ba do not alter the noradrenaline content in the brain but do activate tyrosine hydroxylase, it might be assumed that the turnover of noradrenaline is enhanced under the influence of 30,803-Ba. This assumption is supported by the fact that combined treatment with 30,803-Ba and with the powerful tyrosine-hydroxylase inhibitor alphamethyl tyrosine lowers the content of noradrenaline in the rat brain to a greater extent than treatment with alpha-MT alone[8] and that 30,803-Ba also accelerates the disappearance of intracisternally injected noradrenaline.[7]

It is common knowledge that minor modifications in the chemical structure of a compound may sometimes result in marked changes in its biological activity. I do not know of any other chemical class of compounds in which it would be possible to demonstrate, however, such extreme qualitative variations with regard to the pharmacological effects exerted on such a complex organ as the central nervous system (CNS). There may indeed be reason to assume—by analogy with what we have learned about the peripheral or autonomic synapses with the aid of variations in chemical structure—that such compounds as 30,803-Ba and 34,276-Ba might well help in elucidating the more intimate processes of inhibition or activation occurring within the CNS. This remains to be seen in future investigations.

But now I should like to revert to several questions of a more general nature. In the course of this lecture I have now and again made reference to the term "screening." One sometimes has the impression that the full significance of the term "screening" is not always properly understood, and that here and there the work of screening is regarded as tantamount to an automated, impersonal routine activity. What in fact is meant by screening?

The term "screening" is derived from the word "screen," an instrument originally used in agriculture to separate grains of various sizes. The coarser the sieve, the larger the number of grains that are lost. It is therefore the size of the sieve or, in our case, the fineness of the mesh, that determines how many compounds are retained in the sieve. The comparison with an agricultural instrument, however, is a somewhat lame one, because it is really applicable only to the screening of a single uniform biological function—whereas for the evaluation of a new potential therapeutic agent, which as a rule exerts an influence on the whole organism, what one needs is several qualitatively different "sieves." The choice of mesh is not only a matter of organization but also a question involving imagination and chance, i.e. factors that can be neither learned nor controlled. Screening for the purpose of discovering new therapeutic agents can only be successful, moreover, if due consideration is also given to the current state of knowledge reached by the medical and biological sciences.

In principle, there are a number of ways of classifying research. One method of classification draws a distinction between "basic" and "applied" research, basic research being taken to mean investigations pursued for their own sake, as opposed to applied research in which the main emphasis is placed on practical results. This distinction may well apply to certain branches of research and may also be of some value for statistical purposes. It hardly suffices, however, to cover the complexities of present-day scientific activity in the pharmaceutical industry—for the decisive point here is that progress can be achieved only by unremitting efforts to understand how active substances act and by the elucidation of fundamental physiological and pathophysiological mechanisms.

Today a biological assignment can be tackled with any prospect of success only if consideration is given to as many as possible of the problems that it entails. This means that elements of "basic" research also need to be included. In biological-medical research as pursued by the pharmaceutical industry, then, there is no sharply drawn distinction between basic and applied research—a statement that is no doubt equally valid for nonindustrial medical research as well. The crucial difference between academic and industrial research lies rather in the choice of fields investigated.

So far as biological research in industry is concerned, it is of greater relevance to classify projects by reference to their probable duration instead of trying to assign them to pigeonholes labeled "basic" and "applied." In accordance with the "target-consciousness" inherent in industrial activity, the results these projects yield are required to show some practical value.

Thus, the purpose of research in the pharmaceutical industry can be defined in simple terms: it is to discover drugs. The task of the pharmacologist is to predict the usefulness and safety of a new drug by means of animal experiments. For this purpose, he uses screening tests, which enable him to pick out the active compounds and reject the inactive ones. This screening procedure has several implications: first of all, it involves collaboration with research chemists; this extremely close symbiosis between biology and chemistry, and the genuine partnership that has developed from it, is a salient feature of biological research on an industrial plane.

Moreover, if therapeutic success is to be the ultimate goal, it follows that both biology and chemistry are lost without clinical research. Collaboration with clinical research, however, must be of a very active type, and it must be positively motivated by the clinician's desire to contribute, through the findings he obtains, to the creation of something better. It is in this respect that the kind of clinical research I have in mind differs fundamentally from clinical research undertaken merely in order to comply with certain regulations. The new class of centrally acting substances to which I have just been referring provides a good example in point: it was in fact a clinician who, having been stimulated by the findings we had obtained in our studies with this class of compounds, suggested that clinical trials be carried out with Preparation CIBA 34,276-Ba [5]; his name is Professor Kuhn.

I can still remember, as if it were only yesterday, a discussion that took place within our circle of research workers some 20 years ago, just after reserpine had been isolated in crystalline form. During the discussion, doubts were voiced whether it would be possible to make this reserpine available for clinical trials—the commercialization of the preparation being regarded at that time as inconceivable; these doubts were reinforced by calculations showing that the quantities of substance available were extremely limited and that the cost even of a tablet containing less than 1 mg reserpine would be prohibitive.

The story of how production capacity for the manufacture of reserpine was created reads like a novel and is one that I find even more intriguing than that of the drug's isolation. Owing to the relatively low yield of reserpine from the rauwolfia roots initially available, as well as to certain difficulties of a political nature, CIBA was compelled to conduct throughout the world—in literally the whole of the subtropical and tropical belt in which the rauwolfia plant occurs—a search for species of rauwolfia suitable for manufacturing purposes, to organize expeditions all over the globe, and to set up plantations on an experimental basis. These efforts, moreover, were already undertaken at a time when it was not yet even possible to commence clinical trials on anything approaching a large scale.

Reference is frequently made to the fact that teamwork is of cardinal importance in modern pharmaceutical science; those less familiar with this branch of science, however, often fail to realize that not only collaboration between the laboratory-oriented chemist and biologist, but also collaboration between the latter and the groups responsible for production and pharmaceutical development may likewise be a decisive factor, and that in the last analysis the pharmaceutical industry, too, is one in which there can be no progress where there is no willingness and readiness to run risks and make decisions.

For his valuable help in preparing the English version of this paper, the author wishes to express his sincerest thanks to Mr. H. D. Philps (M. A. Cantab.). He also wishes to thank Prof. M. Staehelin and Dr. L. Maître for kindly providing him with the results of their studies with CIBA 34,276-Ba in the field of catecholamine metabolism.

REFERENCES

1. Bein, H. J.: Pharmacol Rev *8*:435, 1956.
2. ——: *In* Anxiety and Tension—New Therapeutic Aspects, an International Symposium, St. Moritz, January 16, 1970, ed. by Ciba Limited, Basel, Switzerland.
3. Carlsson, A., and Hillarp, N.-A.: Kgl Fysiograf Sallskap Lund Forh *26*:1, 1956.
4. Holzbauer, M., and Vogt, M.: J Neurochem *1*:8, 1956.
5. Kuhn, R.: *In* Cerletti, A., and Bové, F. J., eds.: The Present Status of Psychotropic Drugs, Amsterdam, Excerpta Medical Foundation, 1969, p. 512.
6. Lorez, H.-P.: Z Ges Exp Med *151*:241, 1969.
7. Maître, L., Staehelin, M., and Bein, H. J.: To be published in 1970.
8. Maître, L.: Unpublished results.
9. Müller, J. M., Schlittler, E., and Bein, H. J.: Experientia *8*:338, 1952.
10. Pletscher, A., Shore, P. A., and Brodie, B. B.: Science *122*:374, 1955.
11. Rieppel, F. W.: Deutsch Med Wschr *80*:653, 1955.
12. Wilhelm, M., and Schmidt, P.: Helv Chim Acta *52*:1385, 1969.

CHAPTER 12

Introduction of Neuroleptic Chemotherapy Into Psychiatry

PIERRE DENIKER, MD *

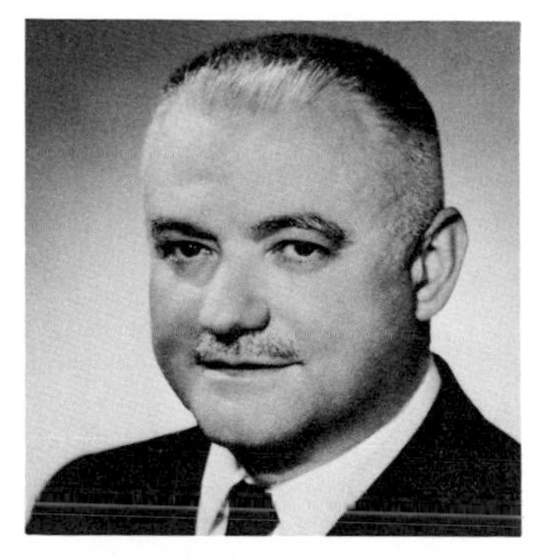

MEDICAL DISCOVERIES are frequently attributed to chance, luck, or even error. In our case, progress might be more accurately attributed to the synthesis of new compounds serving the hypothesis that it is possible to treat mental disorders in a strictly medical sense.

BEFORE CHLORPROMAZINE

Twenty years ago, such an idea might have seemed unrealistic, since, even today, there are psychiatrists who think it impossible to act on the mind by means other than the spoken word. Even before 1952, when chlorpromazine was introduced, several fundamental advances had been made in treating psychoses. They included electroshock or shock induced by fever, Metrazol, or insulin, which are nonspecific therapies or medications, like antibiotics for the treatment of syphilis, affecting the etiological agent rather than the resulting disorders. However, definite etiologies are not known for most psychoses.

The quest for knowledge was as marked 20 years ago as it is today. This was evidenced by the first World Psychiatric Congress held in Paris in 1950. Certain trends among the many quite "unsophisticated" research efforts led to the discovery of modern chemotherapy. Initial studies attempted to analyze the mechanism of

* Professor agrégé, Clinique des Maladies Mentales et de l'Encéphale, Paris.

action of shock therapy. Thus, our first communication on chlorpromazine was presented at the centennial of the French Medico-Psychological Society, which covered shock therapy methods. Jean Delay reviewed them in the light of his studies on the common effects of these different methods on diencephalic centers. Accordingly, they resembled Selye's alarm reaction. This explains our immediate interest in "artificial hibernation," developed by my friend Laborit, because it acts on the mechanisms and structures affected by shock therapy. However, the method we proposed, together with Jean Delay and J. M. Harl,† employed neither hibernation nor sleep therapy.

Another research trend involved attempts to find psychiatric applications for new drugs introduced into general therapy: for instance, the use of procaine and procainamide ‡ for the treatment of hallucinatory psychoses, and, in particular, trials with new antihistamines such as the American investigations with diphenhydramine and the French work with promethazine, a percursor of chlorpromazine. Studies on compounds modifying the nerve cell, such as dinitriles, or application of the psychic effects of certain drugs in psychiatry were also included. For example, by 1952, isoniazid-induced psychic stimulation in tubercular patients led to the use of this iproniazid precursor in depressions.

Although producing more or less negative results, other research contributed to progress by preventing further work in certain fields. For example, the use of opiates and belladonna derivatives, bromides and chloral hydrate, paraldehyde and barbiturates resulted in as many disappointments as hopes. Sleep treatments induce only prolonged sleep whether they are deep narcotherapies, which were developed in Switzerland in 1930, or "conditioned" sleep therapies inspired by Pavlovian ideas. Their indications are neuroses and psychosomatic disorders rather than psychoses.

Drugs with new activity were quickly recognized because of familiarity with available agents. The "lytic cocktail" developed by Laborit combined three drugs: pethidine, a morphine-like derivative; promethazine, an antihistamine; and chlorpromazine. Psychiatrists knew the first two; therefore, interest centered on the last.

† Before his premature death in a mountain accident, he was an intern in our department.

‡ These attempts precede the introduction of substituted benzamides as neuroleptics by 20 years.

CHLORPROMAZINE

In 1950, Charpentier at Rhône Poulenc Laboratories synthesized this phenothiazine, which is related to antiparkinsonian agents and antihistamines. It might still be sitting on the shelf of some chemical laboratory if Laborit had not sought a compound with more central effects than promethazine. With chlorpromazine, he actually reproduced in warm-blooded animals conditions existing in cold-blooded or hibernating ones. However, the possibility seemed remote that the drug might produce in humans the cold-bloodedness, "indifference," or ataraxia extolled by the Stoics. It was Laborit who predicted that the new agent would be used in psychiatry. His colleagues, psychiatrists at the military hospital of Val De Grâce, tried his drug mixture in manic patients. They found its effects interesting but not strong enough and returned to electroshock therapy.

We decided to use the drug without concomitant agents; this may be the first rule of clinical pharmacology. Doses considered high at that time, 75 mg to 150 mg per day, were administered "continuously" in four daily injections. This continuity, which today applies to most psychiatric chemotherapy, was a decisive factor in our success.

Our initial experimental data were very limited. The good pharmacological work of Mrs. Courvoisier and Koetschet *et al.*, as well as Dell's experiments with the reticular formation, was published in 1953. We had only received a few typed sheets in 1952. They were a brief summary for the clinician's use and were distributed with the ampules and tablets. It is disturbing to think that certain effects of the drug were observed in humans before being noted in animals.

Despite great progress, psychiatric wards of 20 years ago still included agitated patients who did not respond to common therapeutic procedures. Pinel had eliminated chains, but existing treatments could not abolish straitjackets and cells. If we were to recreate the atmosphere of an agitated ward for our students' instruction, they would laugh or become skeptical just as if a Western were projected in an operating room. Nevertheless, neuroleptic chemotherapy originated in that atmosphere. Logically, a new drug was tried in cases resistant to all existing therapies. We had scarcely treated 10 patients—with all due respect to the fervent adherents of statistics—when our conviction proved correct. It was supported by the sudden, great interest of the nursing personnel, who had always been reserved about innovations.

From May to July 1952, Delay and I published our observations on chlorpromazine. There were only 38 cases, and our data dealt with the therapeutic indications as well as the inherent effects of the drug. Since then, we have learned from others, but have not changed our initial opinion about chlorpromazine in acute psychoses. Manic excitation and, more generally, psychotic agitation, which were often resistant to shock or sleep therapy, immediately became indications of choice. This effect of the drug became noticeable in the wards and, to us, it is still a pharmacodynamic test for neuroleptic activity.

The antipsychotic activity of the drug was also evident in the treatment of mental confusion. It differed from the sedative effects because drugs reducing mental alertness generally aggravate disorders of wakeful consciousness. In contrast, chlorpromazine only had symptomatic effects in depression. Its sedative and hypnotic activity cannot correct underlying depressions. True antidepressants were discovered later by R. Kuhn and N. Kline.

Agitation, aggressiveness, and delusive conditions of schizophrenics improved. Contact with the patients could be reestablished, but deficiency symptoms did not change markedly. We are still of the same opinion. The great international confrontations of 1955 on chlorpromazine and neuroleptics were necessary to affirm their efficacy in chronic psychoses. The first inhibition-releasing effects in schizophrenia were observed following the introduction of new phenothiazines. (This point will be discussed later.)

However, even the first few clinical observations yielded considerable information on the novel central activity of the drug. It affected regulation of body temperature, pulse, and blood pressure, gastrointestinal motility, blood count, etc. But the impact of the most significant finding was not immediately recognized. It was the characteristic psychomotor indifference that chlorpromazine caused in treated subjects. Later, it was classified as akinesia.

After initial trials, specialists were particularly impressed by the potent sedative activity of the drug. It was more marked than that of any known agent, was accompanied by relatively mild hypnotic activity, and caused reversible sleep. This was the real beginning of research on drugs that would soon increase in number and would be referred to as "tranquilizers." Chlorpromazine was characterized by not only its action on mental alertness but also its ability to induce a new, neuropsychic condition related to akinesia. The development of the class of drugs for which we proposed the name "neuroleptics" was based on these findings.

IDENTIFICATION OF NEUROLEPTICS

Until then, our research had required no particular technical skill. Any clinician using the latest therapeutic agent available, observing its effects especially when they were unexpected, and recording physical and psychic changes, was merely doing what an honest physician should do. Further developments proved more interesting by relating classic knowledge to new observations, which makes research more rewarding.

Cardiologists noted that reserpine caused psychic indifference. This finding led us to study the drug after Nathan Kline and at the same time as Weber and Noce *et al.* Using doses 10 times those commonly given in treating arterial hypertension, we reported in 1954, with Delay and Y. Tardieu, several observations on the similarities and differences in the therapeutic effects and inherent actions of reserpine and chlorpromazine. In the same year, Professor Steck of Lausanne made an important observation. He reported that patients treated with either drug may develop syndromes resembling parkinsonism, and that reserpine may cause restlessness and make it impossible for the subjects to remain seated (akathisia). These symptoms were also seen in lethargic encephalitis after World War I.

In 1955, Delay and I proposed that the two drugs with completely different chemical structures be classified under the same name: "neuroleptic," literally: that which takes the neuron. In 1956, a new piperazine phenothiazine, prochlorperazine, was reported to cause strange hysterical attacks both in women suspected of being neurotic and in soldiers during training. We made an important correlation with "hysteriform" conditions, described between 1920 and 1930 as sequelae of lethargic encephalitis. The new drug caused various types of unusual dyskinesia. Roumanian authors, in particular, had previously described it as an extrapyramidal disorder or disease. But the syndrome that we observed appeared upon administration of the compound and disappeared when treatment was discontinued.

It was found that neuroleptics could experimentally reproduce almost all symptoms of lethargic encephalitis. In fact, it would be possible to cause true encephalitis epidemics with the new drugs. Symptoms progressed from reversible somnolence to all types of dyskinesia and hyperkinesia, and finally to parkinsonism. The symptoms seemed reversible on interruption of medication. Like the encephalitis virus, the drugs acted via the mesodiencephalic extrapyramidal centers.

In 1957, we proposed a general definition of neuroleptics based on similarities between compounds then known, which later would include many chemical groups with different structures. In 1958, a sulfamide phenothiazine became available, which caused very marked akinetic, hypertonic, and hyperkinetic syndromes characteristic of postencephalitic symptoms. At the same time, the drug showed marked therapeutic activity even in chronic psychoses.

In the same year, Belgian investigators tested a new compound, haloperidol. It was selected by Laboratoires Janssen because it caused dyskinesia in animals. These authors furnished additional proof that neurological effects were more important than the chemical structure in characterizing the effects of the drug. In 1960, we showed that the fundamental characteristic of neuroleptics was a combination of antipsychotic and essentially neurological effects.

Since then, the class of neuroleptics has increased by several chemical types: the phenothiazines have different effects depending on the structure of their side chains and substituted radicals. Compounds with aliphatic chains, the chlorpromazine type, have sedative activity mainly accompanied by extrapyramidal and especially autonomic effects. Compounds with piperazine chains, the prochlorperazine type, have inhibition-releasing properties and cause very marked dyskinesia. Those with piperidine chains, the thioridazine type, have moderate activity and slight neurological effects, but they cause endocrine-metabolic changes of central origin. Butyrophenones, already quite numerous—thioxanthenes, dibenzothiazepines, substituted benzamides, several piperazine derivatives, etc. —were developed in addition to phenothiazines and reserpine derivatives. As a result, the list of compounds following chlorpromazine continues to grow.

THERAPEUTIC ACTIVITY AND NEUROLOGICAL EFFECTS

We thought it would be possible to establish a relationship between the therapeutic activity of neuroleptics and their ability to cause specific neurological syndromes. This is one of the most controversial aspects of our studies. Generally, agents used for biological treatment in psychiatry are precisely those that cause "therapeutic diseases" of CNS regulatory mechanisms. This applied to fever in malaria therapy, for which Wagner von Jauregg received the Nobel Prize, and to lobotomy, which induces an organic frontal syndrome, for which Egaz Moniz received the same award. It is also true for insulin, which causes coma, as well as Metrazol and electroshock, which induce artificial epileptic seizures. Neuroleptics cause extrapyramidal syndromes, which minor tranquilizers never induce. Similarly, antidepressants have their own neurological effects: the tremor-dysarthria syndrome of the tricyclic compounds and, more generally, the convulsant activity of various agents of this type.

On the other hand, it must also be admitted that neuroleptics may act without causing neurological symptoms. Although the therapeutic activity of chlorpromazine and reserpine was known before their neurological effects, autonomic changes and akinesia were immediately noted. It was then found that all drugs producing the characteristic neurological syndromes had similar antipsychotic activity. In contrast, compounds of the same chemical group that did not cause neurological effects had almost no therapeutic activity in psychoses.

Sound arguments contradict our neurological theory. Chiefly, no relationship has been established between therapeutic activity and the intensity of neurological symptoms, although better results are sometimes obtained when marked neurological syndromes are systematically induced. Neurological symptoms indicate that there are effects on nervous structures, which are probably involved in the therapeutic process, and perhaps also in the pathology of psychoses. Lethargic encephalitis was known to cause syndromes resembling hebephrenia and catatonia. Cases have also been reported where the occurrence of encephalitis during schizophrenia favorably affected the mental disease.

However, present reasoning involves biochemical factors. The greater sensitivity of certain nervous structures to neuroleptics depends on their particular chemical activity. Research in this area is just beginning and clinicians can make their modest contributions. Cazzullo *et al.* showed that adenosine triphosphate, ATP, prevented histological lesions induced in the animal nervous system by very high doses of neuroleptics. We demonstrated in humans that ATP infusions reduced the hypertonic syndrome. This was experimentally confirmed further. Because of the detailed analysis of changes in facial expression and facial muscle tone, we considered the temporal amygdala to be among the centers affected even by weak neuroleptic treatment.

At present, cerebral amine metabolism is of great interest. It is markedly but differently modified by various neuroleptics. The role of these amines in Parkinson's disease is also known. The effects of our drugs may originate in the basal ganglia, where the biogenic amines are highly concentrated. However, modern biochemistry may consider our agents too crude and their effects too massive for them to be analyzed in detail. We have passed from simple therapeutic observations to rudimentary but sound hypotheses about the mechanisms of action. These hypotheses provide, by way of introduction, a valid methodology in the search for new effective drugs.

The recent introduction of long-acting neuroleptics has shown that equivalent and even better therapeutic effects are possible with much lower doses. The drug quantity once used in a single day now suffices for two to three weeks of treatment, because the drug is slowly released. Thus, the question arose about the kinetics of neuroleptic metabolism in the organism and the brain. Pertinent studies are under way.

POSITIVE AND NEGATIVE ASPECTS

Neuroleptic agents are produced in great quantity and are taken by millions of patients. Thus, an evaluation may be attempted. Simple drugs have facilitated extensive therapy in psychiatric institutions where previously only a few patients benefited from active treatment. If those in charge of American mental health are correct, the generalized use of chemical agents, neuroleptics and others, has decisively influenced overcrowded psychiatric hospitals and facilitated more liberal treatment and its continuation under outpatient conditions.

The discovery of chemotherapeutic agents coincided in all developed countries with a movement supporting better institutional organization for the patients' rehabilitation. Paradoxically, someone assumed a certain opposition between chemotherapy and, on the other hand, sociotherapy and psychotherapy. They actually benefit from one another and are inseparable. We only need to know the role and usefulness of each method in terms of saving human life. Chemotherapy is relatively precise, choice among the different agents is delicate, and strict medical control is indispensable. It may have excellent therapeutic effects in chronic psychoses; however, they are basically transitory because relapses occur when medication is interrupted for a few weeks. This shows the significance of the cooperation between the psychiatrist and the family physician, and the importance of adequately informing the patient's everyday contacts.

These drugs are now widely distributed and very cautiously marketed. Thus, it may seem surprising that the originally unsophisticated psychopharmacological research did not cause more accidents or catastrophes. Although such possibilities did arise, they were generally averted. Furthermore, it might have been feared that these drugs, whose action compares with that of encephalitis and parkinsonism, might eventually induce irreversible secondary neurological syndromes. Such effects cannot be denied: it has been known for some years that permanent dyskinesia may occur in patients treated with neuroleptics and drugs with neurological activity. These phenomena must be recognized in time and treated correctly. Also, they are not absolutely irreversible because they can be relieved by treatment with another appropriate neuroleptic. Ocular and dermatological complications have received much attention, especially in America; I am referring to the "purple people." These disorders occurred in patients who received high doses for a very long time without adequate supervision. This finding supports our statements about strict medical control. Finally, in certain predisposed subjects, potent neuroleptics may cause actual "malignant" syndromes with hyperthermia. When discovered in time, they can always be checked by discontinuing the causal agent and using appropriate treatment.

Overall, neuroleptics are more useful than dangerous when treatment is suitably administered and supervised. A more theoretical aspect of the new chemotherapeutic agents is their contribution to the development of a more medically and scientifically oriented psychiatry since their use requires more comprehensive and advanced training for physicians and nursing personnel. Any stimulation of psychiatrists and their collaborators that prompts them to further their medical and psychological knowledge simultaneously expands the future possibilities of our discipline.

Another point should be observed. Almost 20 years ago, a simple drug was found to act directly on a psychopathological process. This finding was very important, although the precise etiology of this process was still unknown. It is now established that mental disorders may be chemically induced, for example pharmacopsychoses, and then relieved by means that are effective in both artificial and natural psychoses. This theory supports the biochemical origin of psychoses.

Neuroleptics are only part of the new field of psychopharmacology in which remarkable discoveries have been made, such as antidepressants. Psychopharmacology has probably existed as long as physicians have been searching for drugs affecting insanity. The introduction of neuroleptics at a crucial time when shock therapy had achieved all its objectives decisively influenced present-day psychiatry. Despite the development of more scientific therapy—the term clinical psychopharmacology is currently used—we must not forget that experimental subjects are human beings suffering from the worst disorders. They are not an anonymous "clinical material" to be treated with questionnaires that are evaluated by computers only.

CHAPTER

13

The Butyrophenone Story

PAUL A. J. JANSSEN, MD *

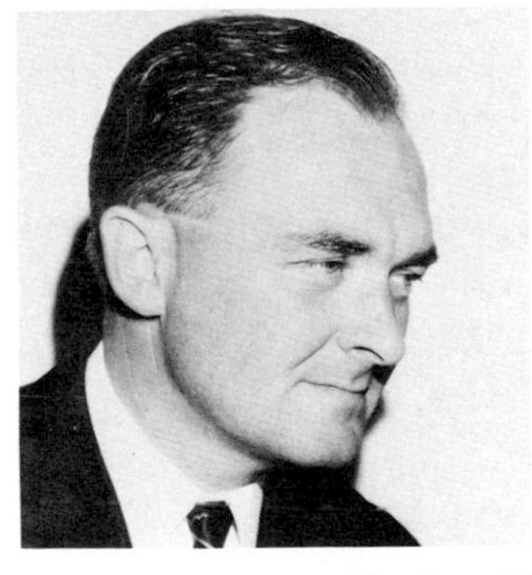

ON JUNE 27 OF LAST YEAR I went to the Beerse laboratory as usual and found on my desk a letter signed by my friend Dr. Frank Ayd, telling me about an international symposium of historical interest to be held at Taylor Manor Hospital in Baltimore in April, 1970, inviting me to attend and tell the story of the butyrophenones, and announcing that I would be one of the recipients of the Taylor Manor Hospital Award as a special tribute for what was said to be an outstanding contribution to the conquest of emotional and mental disorders. I felt pleased, honored, and very grateful. And this mood-elevating effect of Frank's letter was strongly reinforced by the similar elation within my family.

A few days later, however, when starting to plan this manuscript, which I was asked to submit before the end of the year, I started to feel differently. I felt in fact increasingly hesitant and surprisingly confused. When trying to reduce to writing a story that is really part of one's own life, and realizing that it will be read by both insiders and outsiders, one tries to evaluate the pros and cons of different alternative strategic and tactical approaches. Should it be a so-called objective scientific paper, a cold-blooded enumeration of established facts, or should it be a simple human story, emphasizing its psychological and emotional aspects? Would it be possible to come up with an acceptable mixture of these two extremes and still satisfy the suspected requirements of the audience? And, above

* Director, Janssen Pharmaceutica; Beerse, Belgium.

all, is it really possible on an occasion like this to do proper justice to all those who contributed to the development of these drugs: my collaborators at the laboratory and the numerous clinical investigators, particularly those who were willing to help at the very beginning of the butyrophenone story? Today is January 2, 1970. I am still considering the pros and cons, but now the story must be written without further delay. Frank is waiting. The open mind of course never acts. So let me close my eyes and jump, because who wants to die intestate?

After I was graduated from the University of Ghent in 1951, I was drafted and spent 18 months as a military physician with the Belgian army in Germany. Duties were extremely light. There was plenty of time to think, to study medicinal chemistry and pharmacology as well as to plan for the future. Thanks to the courtesy of Professor J. Schueller, I was able to use the laboratory and library facilities of the pharmacological department of Cologne University daily and almost full-time.

When the army sent me to my Belgian hometown Turnhout to finish the last four months of military service, I had made up my mind. In 1935, my father, Constant Janssen, after 12 years of medical practice, had founded a pharmaceutical company, which, in 1953, was manufacturing an astonishing variety of classic ethical prescription drugs and selling them primarily in Belgium. The family enterprise was relatively successful but had no research, no chemical manufacturing, no patents, and therefore little hope for eventual expansion in other markets. What the company needed were better, original and patentable products. The answer to its problems, I felt strongly, was efficient research. The odds against success were apparently enormous. The available laboratory space was a small section of the existing analytical quality control laboratory. Trained personnel was virtually nonexistent and so was the budget. The only way out was somehow to try to concentrate on making new chemicals that could be synthesized and purified with simple methods and equipment, using the cheapest possible intermediates, and efficiently investigated pharmacologically at minimal expense (Fig. 1). The fact that the oldest member of our very small research group was 27 years of age, that we were all willing to work very long hours, seven days a week, and, being inexperienced, had no idea of the difficulties along the road but blind faith in ultimate success, were of course decisive factors in our favor.

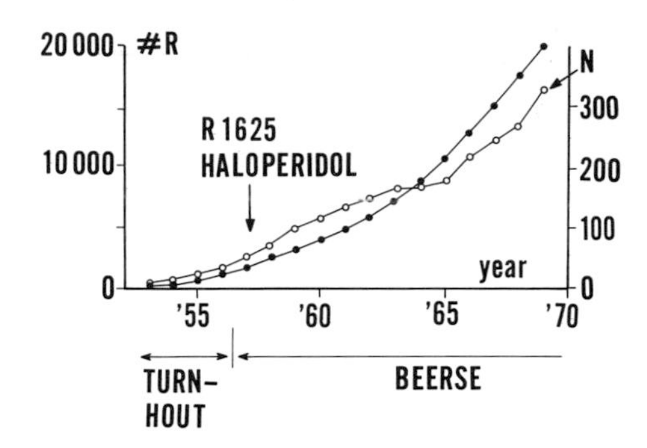

Size (N) of the research team (○—○) and number of new compounds (#R, sequence number) synthesized at Janssen Pharmaceutica at the end of each year. (1953–1969).

Our first patents were filed in 1954, and started to create financial return in 1955. In 1957 we moved from the Turnhout factory into the newly built research laboratories in Beerse, a few miles west of Turnhout on the road to Antwerp. By then, of course, the research team had grown to about 50 people, and we built small but efficient laboratories as well as the first pilot plant and better animal quarters. We had synthesized and screened well over 1,000 new molecules, which are referred to as "Research-" or "R-products," and our first important drug, the anticholinergic compound isopropamide or R 79, was enjoying its first successful year of trade. Royalty income from our licensees was increasing and enabled us to do more research.

The first butyrophenone derivative of interest we discovered in 1957, a few months after we resettled in Beerse. We were increasingly interested by then, as we are today, in trying to understand better the relationship between chemical structure and physicochemical properties on the one hand, and pharmacological effects, the interaction of synthetic molecules with living matter, on the other hand. This type of knowledge, I thought, was likely to improve our batting average and would eventually lead to tailor-made drugs with predictable predetermined biological properties. We could at any rate not conceive of any faster or more efficient way to reach our goals.

In 1954 we had applied this strategy to the study of 3:3-diphenylpropylamines and it had produced the long-acting anticholinergic drug isopropamide (R 79) and the powerful narcotic analgesic dextromoramide (R 875). A similar systematic study of 4-phenylpiperidines related to pethidine produced in 1956 the first synthetic specific antidiarrheal agent diphenoxylate (R 1132) as well as serial number R 951, a propiophenone derived, by Mannich reaction, from norpethidine and acetophenone (Fig. 2). We were quite excited about the very high order of morphinomimetic potency of this propiophenone and started to examine the effect of systematic structural changes on potency. One of these modifications consisted in lengthening the two-carbon chain linking the basic nitrogen to the ketonic carbon atom, thus producing a butyrophenone derivative of norpethidine, R 1187. When this new chemical was injected in mice, a behavioral effect reminiscent of both morphine and chlorpromazine was observed. Immediately after the dose, the ani-

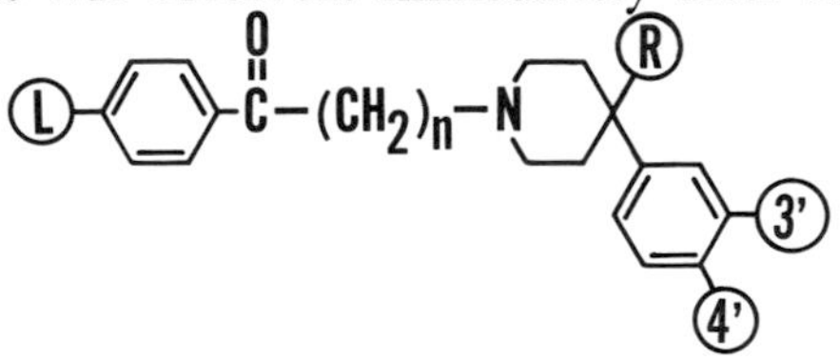

R	n	L	4'	3'		activity: morphine–like	activity: chlorpromazine–like
$COOC_2H_5$	2	H	H	H	R 951	+++	o
$COOC_2H_5$	3	H	H	H	R 1187	++	+
OH	3	H	H	H	R 1472	o	++
OH	3	F	H	H	R 1589 peridol	o	+++
OH	3	F	Cl	H	R 1625 haloperidol	o	++++
OH	3	F	CH_3	H	R 1658 methylperidol	o	++++
OH	3	F	H	CF_3	R 2498 trifluperidol	o	++++
					morphine	++	o
					pethidine	+	o
					chlorpromazine	o	++

mals showed morphine-like excitement, mydriasis and insensitivity to noxious stimuli, but subsequently they became progressively calm, sedated and slightly catatonic. This was a great day in the laboratory. In 1957 of course only the rauwolfia alkaloid reserpine and a few phenothiazine derivates related to chlorpromazine were known to be useful as neuroleptic drugs or major tranquilizers for the treatment of psychomotor agitation as observed in a variety of mental illnesses, including schizophrenia and mania.

From the point of view of its chemical structure, apparently unrelated to the known major tranquilizers, the chlorpromazine-like activity of the butyrophenone derived from norpethidine thus came as a great surprise. However, this prototype R 1187 was not thought to be of any particular practical interest, because of its mixed morphine-like and chlorpromazine-like properties and because it was, like chlorpromazine, active only at relatively high dose levels. It was therefore immediately decided to synthesize related molecules in order to get rid of the morphine-like effect and to increase both neuroleptic potency and specificity. Within a short time we found that the replacement of the ester moiety of the prototype R 1187 by a tertiary alcohol group produced a 4-phenyl-4-piperidinol-butyrophenone, R 1472, which brought us much closer to our goal. This aminoalcohol was indeed completely devoid of morphinomimetic effects and almost indistinguishable from chlorpromazine in its pharmacological profile.

It was then learned that certain aromatic substituents on the two aromatic rings of R 1472 had a striking potency-increasing effect and also increased duration of action. Several hundreds of related molecules were prepared and pharmacologically investigated until, early in 1958, I was convinced that we had several new molecules available that would merit clinical testing. The most potent, longest-acting and most specific neuroleptic of the series was serial number R 1625, derived from 4-fluorobutyrophenone and 4-(4'-chlorophenyl)-piperidin-4-ol (Fig. 3). R 1625, or haloperidol, was by far the most active neuroleptic drug known in 1958. It was many times more potent than chlorpromazine, was both faster- and longer-acting, was as potent orally as parenterally, was chemically pure, soluble and stable in aqueous solution, was almost devoid of the antiadrenergic and other autonomic effects of chlorpromazine, had a more favorable safety ratio, and was surprisingly well tolerated when given chronically to laboratory animals.

All these findings convinced us that we had a drug in our hands

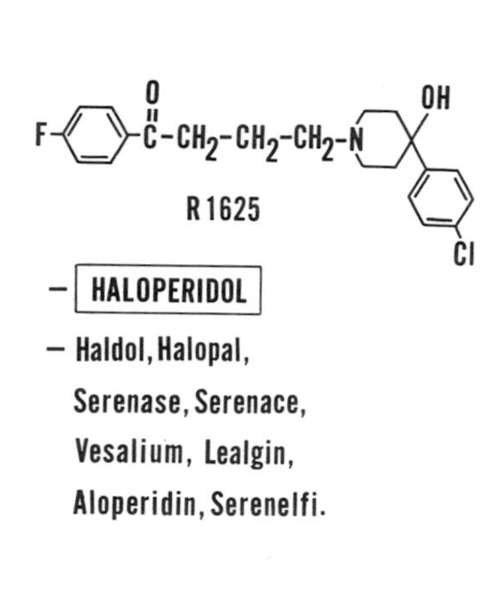

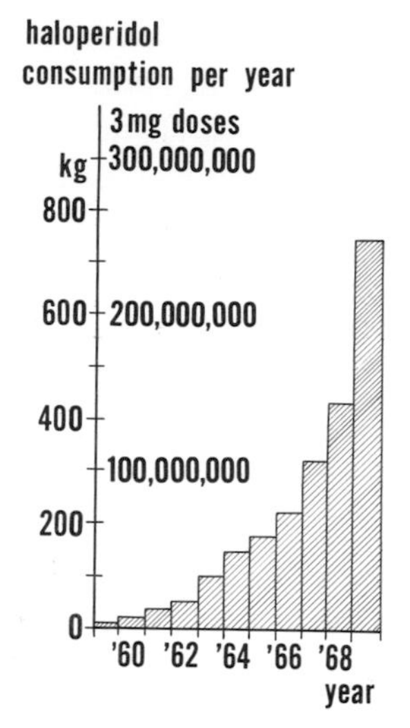

Quantity of haloperidol consumed for medical purposes between 1959 and the end of 1969: 2260 kg or 753,000,000 daily doses of 3 mg.

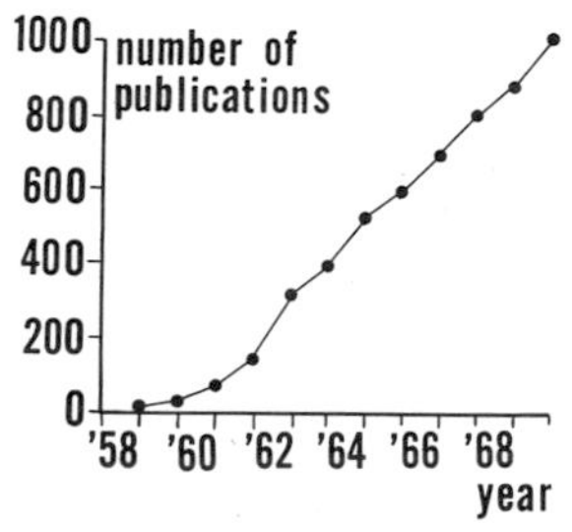

Over 1000 scientific papers on haloperidol published between 1958 and 1969.

that would probably produce chlorpromazine-like effects in the clinic but was likely to do so at 50 to 100 times lower dose levels. I also remember being greatly impressed with the fact that, in rats, haloperidol is a much more specific antagonist of amphetamine than chlorpromazine, because amphetamine intoxication was known to induce a psychiatric syndrome in man that is often almost indistinguishable from paranoid psychosis. From these animal studies we predicted that a single parenteral or oral dose of about 5 mg of haloperidol would be both active and safe in the psychotic adult. We therefore decided to prepare haloperidol ampules containing 5 mg per ml and started looking for a psychiatrist willing to start trying these ampules in patients with severe psychomotor agitation.

Within a few weeks the first such patients were being treated with intravenous doses of haloperidol at the psychiatric clinic of Liege University by P. Divry, J. Bobon, J. Collard, A. Pinchard and E. Nols. In October, 1958, the first results of this pilot trial were presented at a meeting of the Belgian Society for Mental Diseases in Brussels and subsequently published in *Acta Neurologica et Psychiatrica Belgica.* This original paper describes the effects of 100 intravenous doses of 2 to 5 mg of haloperidol in a heterogenous group of 18 patients of all ages suffering from severe psychomotor agitation of psychotic, neurotic and psychopathic origin. The drug was said to be obviously and highly effective as a psychomotor sedative within 5 to 15 minutes and for about 3 to 5 hours. Tolerance was excellent. The hypnotic effect of barbiturates was potentiated. Haloperidol was the drug of choice in the emergency treatment of psychomotor agitation independent of its etiology.

Even today, almost 12 years later, this is still a remarkable publication. The experiment was uncontrolled, the data very limited both in number and in time, and yet the conclusions remain as valid today as they were in 1958. There can be little doubt that this and subsequent clinical pilot studies in Liege are historically of essential importance in the development of the butyrophenone series, and I am happy to be able on this occasion publicly to express my feelings of great gratitude to J. Bobon and his collaborators.

By the end of 1958, a rapidly increasing number of clinical trials with haloperidol had been organized in Western Europe, particularly in Belgium, France, Germany, Denmark, Sweden, Spain, Italy Portugal, Switzerland, Finland and Turkey, and on September 5, 1959, 45 psychiatrists, psychologists, neurologists, anesthesiologists and pharmacologists from these 11 countries attended the first international symposium on haloperidol in Beerse in order to present and discuss 17 papers on the subject. It was a truly remarkable day because most of what can be said today about the clinical effects of haloperidol was already recognized and largely agreed on: its usefulness in the treatment of psychomotor agitation in general, hallucinations, manic symptoms, paranoid ideation and delusions, choreic movements and tics, aggressive and impulsive tendencies in psychopaths, certain forms of anxiety and insomnia, nausea and vomiting, and in general all those psychiatric symptoms that are generally recognized today as good indications for neuroleptic therapy. Its neurological side-effect liability was described in detail and the useful doses were said to range from 1 to 15 mg daily, both orally and parenterally.

Particularly gratifying to all participants of the haloperidol research program was the clinical report presented by J. Delay, P. Pichot, Miss Lemperiere and B. Elissalde from the Sainte Anne Clinique in Paris, where chlorpromazine and several other phenothiazines had been originally tested. In this paper the statement was made that the therapeutic results with haloperidol are generally superior to those obtainable with all other neuroleptic drugs, remarkable in manic states and in acute delirium, satisfactory in acute schizophrenia and in chronic delirium, disappointing in hebephrenic patients. The anxiety in melancholia was said to disappear, while the depression remained unaltered.

A month after the symposium in Beerse, haloperidol was made available to the Belgian psychiatric profession and within two years the drug was being prescribed in most Western European countries. The end of 1969 marked the tenth anniversary of the introduction of haloperidol in medical practice. In these ten years, its acceptance by the profession has been steadily growing, particularly since 1967. We remember these years primarily as a strenuous uphill battle. Of the 2,260 kg representing 753,000,000 daily 3 mg doses of haloperidol prescribed in this period, about one half was used over the past two years. In 1969 the drug was available in almost all countries of the world, and today at least 1,000,000 mental patients are being treated with haloperidol.

Its main use remains the treatment of a variety of mental diseases in both ambulatory and hospitalized patients, but haloperidol is also increasingly being used in neurology, anesthesiology, radiotherapy, internal medicine, particularly gastroenterology and obstetrics, as well as in veterinary practice. Between 1958 and 1969, over 1,000 scientific publications on haloperidol appeared in the literature, 80% on clinical results and 20% on pharmacological, chemical, biochemical and pharmaceutical aspects.

In recent years, our own work on haloperidol has been primarily concerned with problems of theoretical interest, such as its metabolism and its mechanism of action. Most gratifying is the fact that the old dream with which it all started is becoming more of a reality: based on the accumulated knowledge in the field of chemical structure-neuroleptic activity relationships, the design of new tailor-made drugs of this type has become a fascinating intellectual game, opening a whole new world full of realistic probabilities and possibilities that will occupy many generations to come. In many other laboratories as well, haloperidol is increasingly being used as a scientific tool for the further exploration of various biochemical and physiological problems related to the function of the brain.

The discovery of the first neuroleptically active butyrophenone in 1957 and of the subsequent clinical development of haloperidol was followed by a period of increasing research and development activity in many laboratories. Well over 5,000 organic bases related to haloperidol have since been prepared and pharmacologically investigated, about 4,000 of them in our own laboratories in Beerse. Over 100 patents describing various butyrophenones have been applied for and this number is increasing day after day. At least 25 of these compounds underwent clinical trial and 10 of them are now being used as drugs in human and in veterinary medicine. Our own research effort led to the clinical trial of 17 of these clinically tested butyrophenones, of which the following 9 are now commercially available for clinical and/or veterinary use:

haloperidol (R 1625)	introduced in 1959
fluanisone (R 2028)	introduced in 1960
trifluperidol (R 2498)	introduced in 1961
pipamperone (R 3345)	introduced in 1961
moperone (R 1658)	introduced in 1963
droperidol (R 4749)	introduced in 1963
benperidol (R 4584)	introduced in 1965
azaperone (R 1929)	introduced in 1968
spiperone (R 5147)	introduced in 1969

Each of these drugs has its own particular pharmacological spectrum of properties and consequently its own special indications. Chemically they are all derived from p-fluoro-butyrophenone. Haloperidol, moperone and trifluperidol are derived from 4-phenylpiperidine, spiperone, droperidol and benperidol from 4-anilinopiperidine, pipamperone from 4-piperidinopiperidine, fluanisone and azaperone from a 4-arylpiperazine. Most of these butyrophenones are primarily intended for psychiatric prescription, but droperidol is mainly used by anesthesiologists and azaperone exclusively in

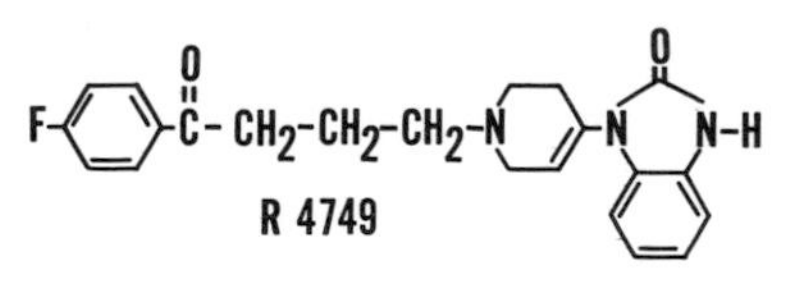

– DROPERIDOL

– Dehydrobenzperidol, Inapsin, Droleptan, Dridol, Leptanal, Leptofen, Innovar, Innovar-vet, Thalamonal.

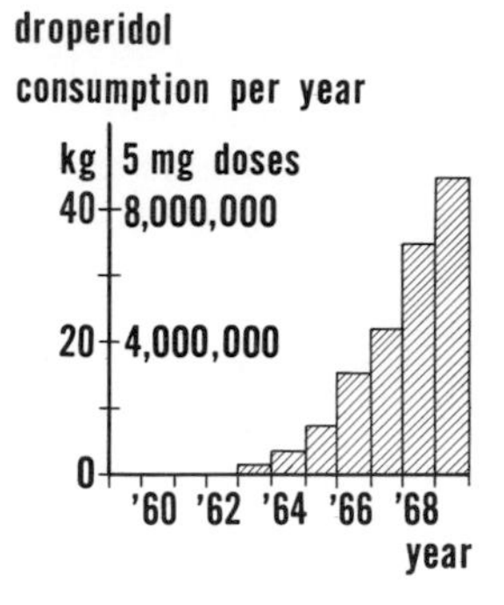

– Quantity of droperidol consumed for medical and veterinary purposes between 1963 and 1969: 130 kg or 26,000,000 single doses of 5 mg.
– 710 scientific papers on droperidol published between 1962 and 1969.

R 4263

FENTANYL

component of Innovar and Thalamonal.

veterinary medicine. To tell the detailed story of every one of these drugs would of course keep us busy much too long, so let me rather select a few examples at random.

Droperidol (R 4749) (Fig. 4) was the result of a long period of research for a potent, very fast, short-acting and well-tolerated neuroleptic drug with pronounced antishock and antiemetic activity. There appeared to be a great need in anesthesiology for a major tranquilizer of this type. The first pilot study in anesthesiology, carried out in 1961 at the University of Brussels by J. De Castro and P. Mundeleer, confirmed the predictions from animal testing. In man a parenteral dose of 5 mg rapidly produces a desirable state of tranquility and detachment without loss of consciousness. Environment-induced anxiety disappears. Voluntary movements are rare, while the patient remains cooperative. Droperidol is extremely effective against cardiac, traumatic and hemorrhagic shock, both prophylactically and therapeutically. It prevents post-operative nausea and vomiting. The use of droperidol in anesthesiologic practice is increasing rapidly in virtually all countries of the world, including the USA and USSR, particularly in combination with the most powerful, fastest- and shortest-acting analgesic known, fentanyl (R 4263), which was also discovered in our laboratories in 1961.

In recent years, droperidol was found to be of great use in many other circumstances. Bobon and collaborators in Liege found the drug to be the fastest and most potent agent known for treating extremely agitated patients. Its ability almost immediately to stop a typical attack of Menière's disease is attracting increasing interest among otorhinolaryngologists.

The antishock effectiveness of droperidol can save many lives, not only in anesthesiology, but also in cardiology for the treatment of cardiac shock associated with myocardial infarction and in the treatment of traumatic and hemorrhagic shock. A collaborative study by several university hospitals in Holland recently showed droperidol to be suprisingly helpful in the treatment of patients with intractable chronic pain and with psychic-dependence problems related to alcohol- and narcotics-addiction.

Ever since Dr. R. Marsboom joined our research team in 1960, after a successful career as a veterinarian in Africa, veterinary research in Beerse has been increasing. As a result, interesting uses for droperidol in animals were discovered. The most interesting probably is the fact that captive gorillas, chimpanzees and orang-outangs will readily drink milk containing droperidol. After a few minutes, the otherwise dangerous and untractable ape will be in a typical catatonic state and readily allow himself to be handled. Previously impractical surgical and diagnostic interventions can thus be carried out with great ease.

One surprising fact about tranquilizers in veterinary practice is their amazing species specificity, which generally limits the usefulness of a particular drug to a few species only, particularly when the requirements are equally specific. A systematic screening effort in this field led to the development of fluanisone (R 2028) (Fig. 5) as a specific tranquilizer for poultry and of azaperone (R 1929), the tranquilizer of choice in pigs and a variety of wild animals. Azaperone has been shown to be of great economical significance in the pig industry because of its ability to prevent

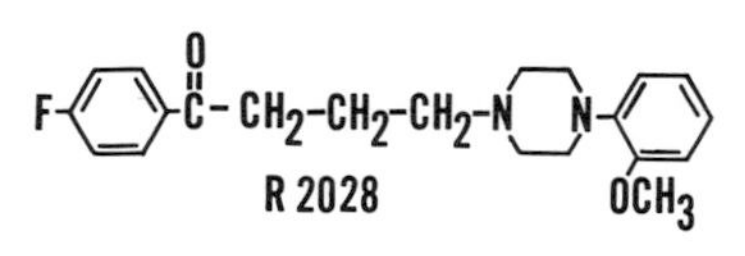

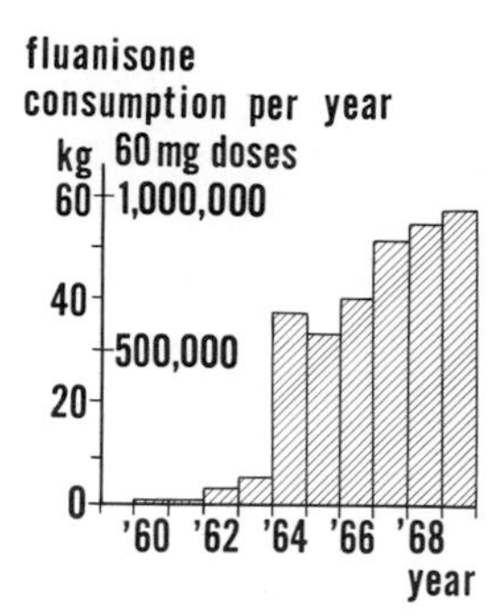

— FLUANISONE

— Haloanisone, Sedalande, Hypnorm, Companin, Anti–picca, Solusediv.

— Quantity of fluanisone consumed for medical and veterinary purposes between 1960 and 1969: 285 kg or 4,750,000 daily doses of 60 mg.

— 150 scientific papers on fluanisone published between 1960 and 1969.

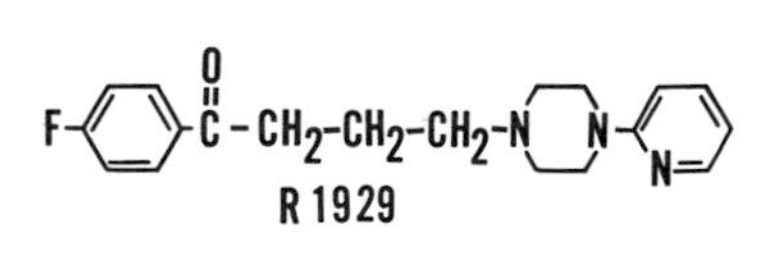

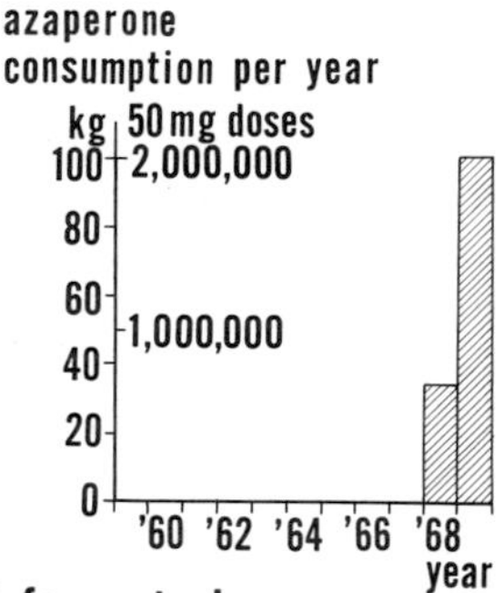

— AZAPERONE

— Stresnil, Eucalmyl, Azaperone—vet.

— Quantity of azaperone consumed for veterinary purposes between 1968 and 1969: 134 kg or 2,680,000 single doses of 50 mg.

— 16 scientific papers on azaperone published between 1967 and 1969.

dramatically the losses induced by various forms of stress and aggressive behavior. In South Africa and in Rhodesia, particularly, Pienaar and others developed interesting techniques for immobilizing and capturing many species of wild animals more safely than ever possible before the azaperone era.

Trifluperidol (R 2498) (Fig. 6) was synthesized in the period when haloperidol (R 1625) was already undergoing clinical trial. It was also brought to the clinic primarily because of its high potency in animals. In man, trifluperidol resembles haloperidol in most respects, but the average useful dose is 2 to 3 times lower. In

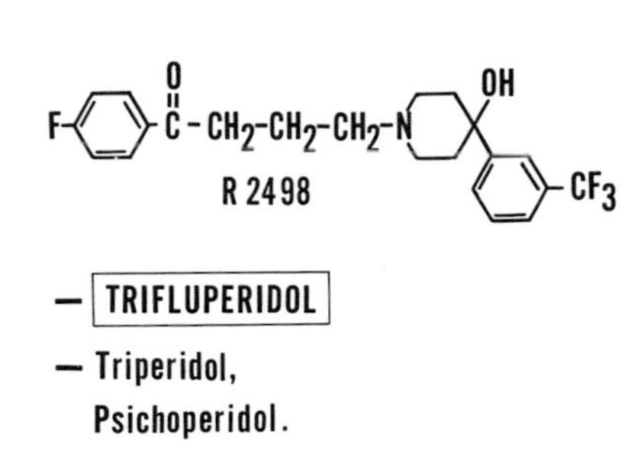

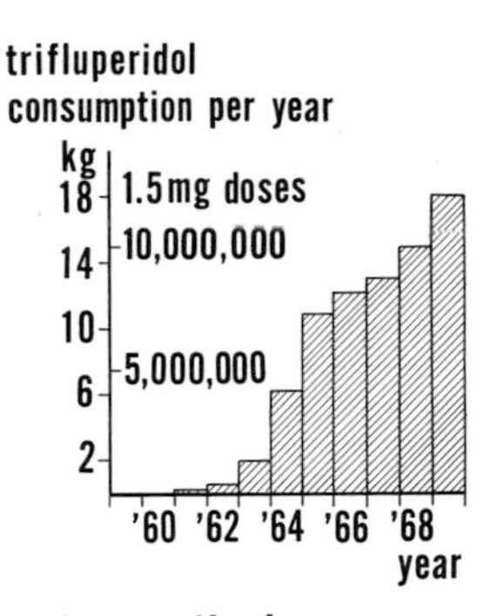

— Quantity of trifluperidol consumed for medical purposes between 1961 and 1969:
77.6 kg or 51,700,000 daily doses of 1.5 mg.

— 200 scientific papers on trifluperidol published between 1960 and 1969.

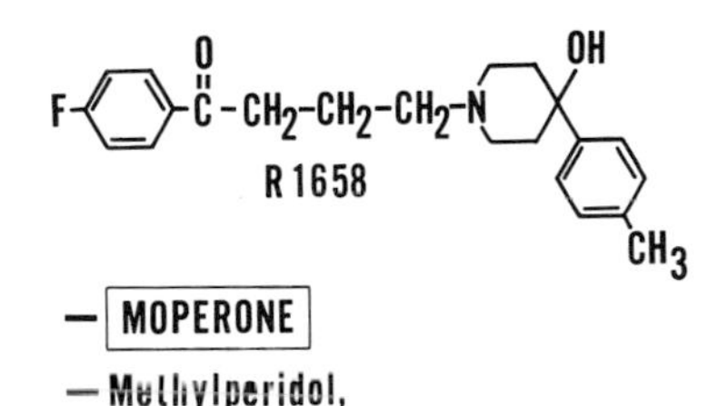

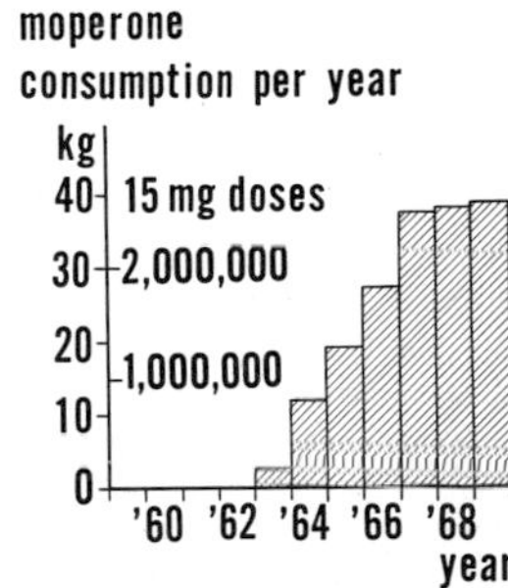

— Quantity of moperone consumed for medical purposes between 1963 and 1969:
171 kg or 11,400,000 daily doses of 15 mg.

— 40 scientific papers on moperone published between 1959 and 1969.

several controlled trials, trifluperidol showed up significantly better than the phenothiazine derivatives with which it was compared, particularly in withdrawn, autistic schizophrenic patients. In clinical practice, moperone was found an effective neuroleptic drug and surprisingly free of side effects when given on a t.i.d. schedule for maintenance therapy in schizophrenia. In severe cases, however, particularly those that apparently need a relatively constant and pronounced neuroleptic effect, day and night, moperone might not be sufficiently effective unless given at impractically frequent intervals.

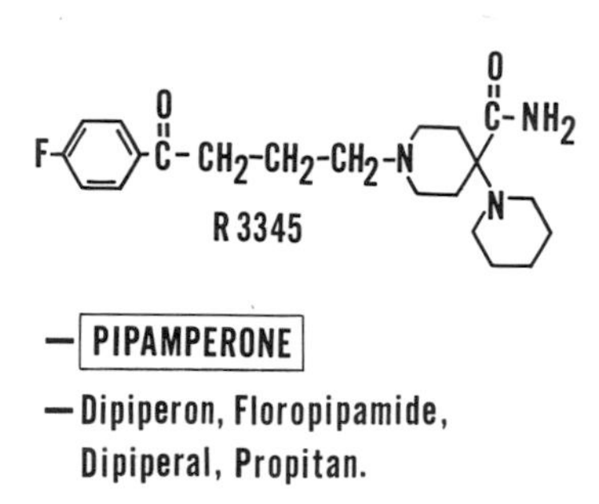

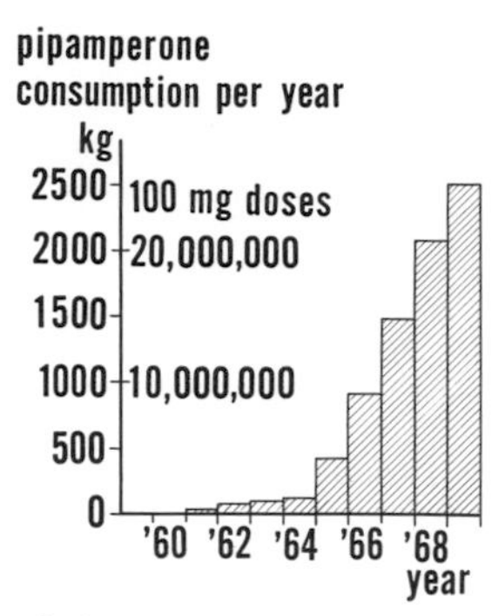

—Quantity of pipamperone consumed for medical purposes between 1961 and 1969: 7760 kg or 77,600,000 daily doses of 100 mg.

—75 scientific papers on pipamperone published between 1961 and 1969.

Pipamperone (Dipiperone or R 3345) (Fig. 7) aroused our interest in 1960 because of its very peculiar pharmacological spectrum. At high dose levels, it acts like many other neuroleptic drugs, but, unlike any other clinically used drug known, it showed itself capable of antagonizing tryptamine seizures at low dose levels. It also has unique taming effects in the aggressive monkey. The first clinical studies showed pipamperone to be different from the known psychopharmaceuticals, both in its effects and in its side effect liability. It has a normalizing effect on mood and on disturbed sleep patterns. Pipamperone is of particular interest in the treatment of various psychopathic syndromes such as destructive, explosive and belligerent tendencies, e.g., in delinquents.

Benperidol (R 4584) and spiperone (R 5147) (Fig. 8) are, on a weight basis, by far the most active neuroleptics used in medical practice, the active daily maintenance dose ranging from 0.05 mg per adult upwards. Benperidol resembles droperidol both chemically and pharmacologically, but is much longer-acting. One of its most interesting indications is in hospitalized patients with disturbing hypersexual tendencies.

Spiperone was recently introduced in Japan. Its therapeutic effectiveness in many drug-resistant chronic schizophrenics is quite striking.

In closing, I would like to express publicly my deep gratitude to all my friends and collaborators who made possible whatever prog-

R 4584

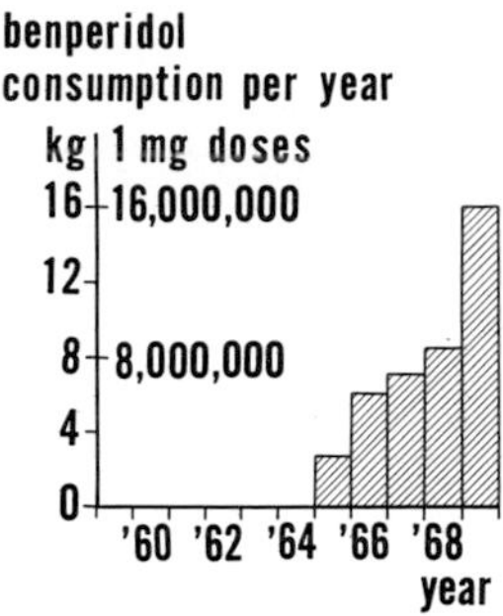

— BENPERIDOL

— Benzperidol, Glianimon, Frenactil, Concilium.

— Quantity of benperidol consumed for medical purposes between 1965 and 1969: 41.2 kg or 41,200,000 daily doses of 1 mg.

— 95 scientific papers on benperidol published between 1962 and 1969.

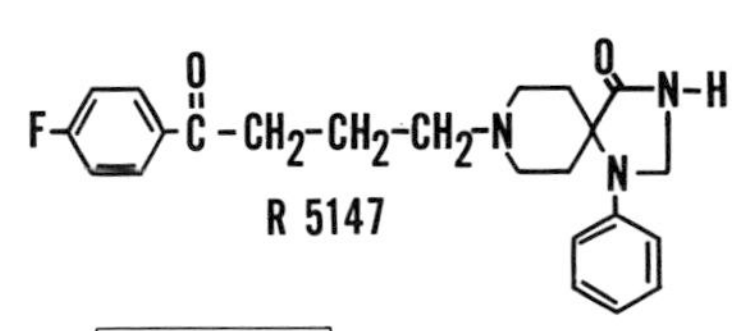

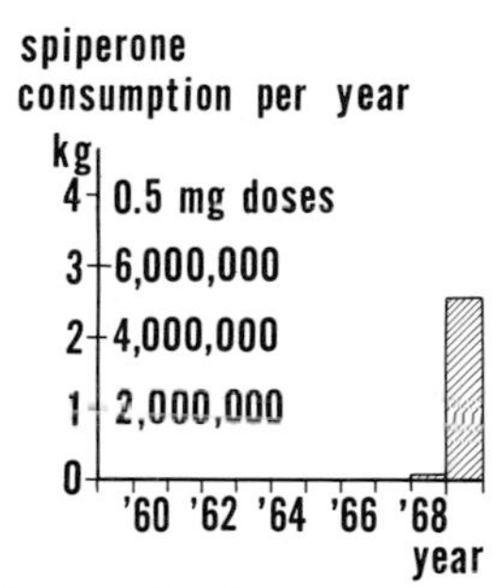

— SPIPERONE

— Spiroperidol, Spiropitan.

— Quantity of spiperone consumed for medical purposes between 1968 and 1969: 2.5 kg or 5,000,000 daily doses of 0.5 mg.

— 30 scientific papers on spiperone published between 1963 and 1969.

ress has been made in discovering and developing the butyrophenones: the organic chemists, the analytical chemists, the pharmacologists, the toxicologists, the biochemists, the statisticians, the clinicians, the coordinators, the instrument builders, the administrators, the secretaries. I thank them not only because of their efforts and intellectual contributions, but above all because they had faith and confidence in the future at a time when faith and confidence were our only assets.

CHAPTER

14

The History of the Thioxanthenes

JØRGEN RAVN, MD, PHD *

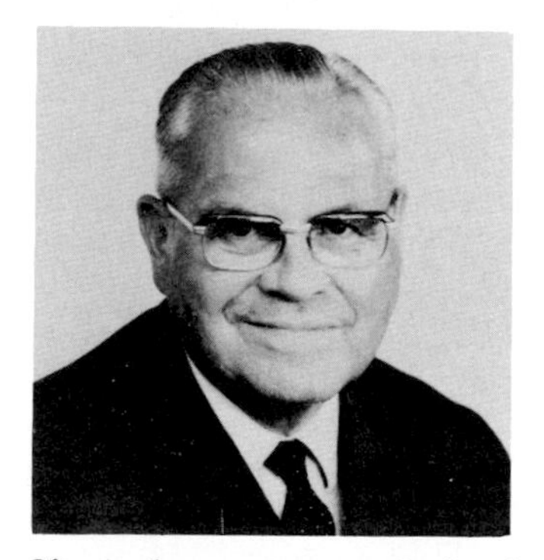

IN THE AUTUMN OF 1958, a research team from the Danish firm H. Lundbeck & Co. suggested to me a clinical trial with a neuroleptic compound, chlorprothixene, representing the first member of a new chemical group, the thioxanthenes. A preliminary clinical trial performed at the Mental Hospital at Middelfart soon disclosed the favorable properties of this compound. Since then, as more derivatives were developed and tested clinically, the thioxanthenes have proved a valuable alternative to the phenothiazine as well as the butyrophenone type of neuroleptic.

I. CHEMISTRY

In July 1958, *P. V. Petersen and co-workers* published the first paper on the chemistry and biological activity of a series of thioxanthenes.[31] The thioxanthene nucleus differs from the phenothiazine nucleus in that the aromatic nitrogen atom is replaced by a

phenothiazine

thioxanthene

FIG. 1.

carbon atom (Fig. 1). In phenothiazine-based neuroleptics such as chlorpromazine, perphenazine and fluphenazine, the basic or amine side chain is attached to the nucleus at the N atom (position 10).

* Head, the Mental Hospital in Middelfart, Department K, Denmark.

Accordingly, the same side chains were attached to the carbon atom in the center ring of the thioxanthene nucleus. It was found that neuroleptic activity was present only in those derivatives where the connection between the side chain and the C_9 carbon atom of the thioxanthene nucleus was established through a double bond.

The first neuroleptic or major tranquilizer of this group to be developed, chlorprothixene, is an analogue of chlorpromazine and accordingly has the following configuration (Fig. 2). Further

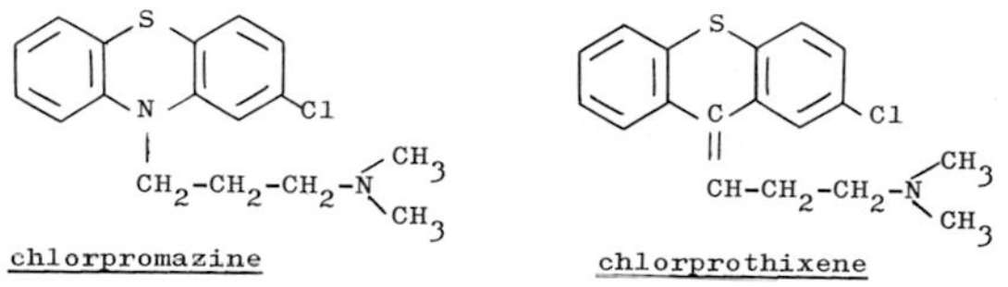

chlorpromazine   chlorprothixene

FIG. 2.

studies of a considerable number of thioxanthene derivatives have shown, not unexpectedly, that the structure-activity relationships of the thioxanthene compounds resemble in many ways those of the corresponding phenothiazine derivatives. Specific for the chemistry of these thioxanthenes is the fact that there exist two isomeric forms of each derivative that has a substituent in one of the phenyl rings. All the derivatives in use have a substituent in position 2: Cl, CF_3 or $SO_2N(CH_3)_2$. The two isomers represent a cis and trans form and the difference is based on the lack of free rotation around the double bond. Taking chlorprothixene as an example, the two isomeric forms may be represented as shown in Figure 3, where

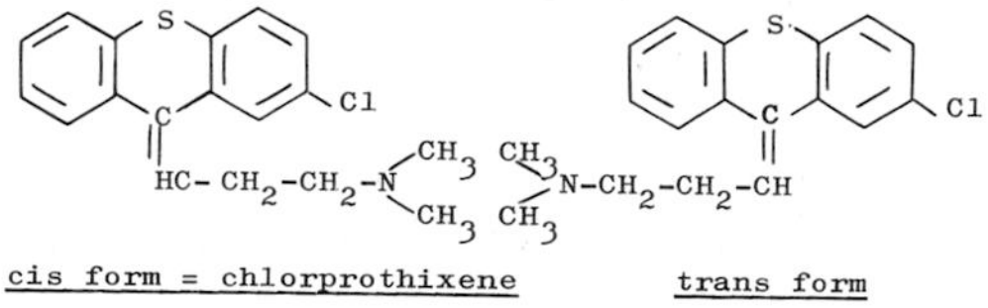

cis form = chlorprothixene   trans form

FIG. 3.

the orientation of the side chain in relation to the chlorine atom represents the difference. Only the cis form shows high central and neuroleptic activity. The active isomer chlorprothixene was, for various reasons, originally designated "trans." X-ray-crystallographic examination, however, has revealed that the active isomer in fact has the cis configuration (*Dunitz et al.*).[8]

The thioxanthene compounds do not show the same sensitivity to UV light as the phenothiazines, which form bluish violet colored products when exposed to sunlight. The metabolites of the thioxanthenes are of course different from those of the phenothiazines. This fact may be the reason why photosensitization and skin pigmentation do not seem to occur as a result of the administration of the thioxanthenes.

The four thioxanthene derivatives that so far are on the market have the following chemical configurations (Fig. 4). It will be seen

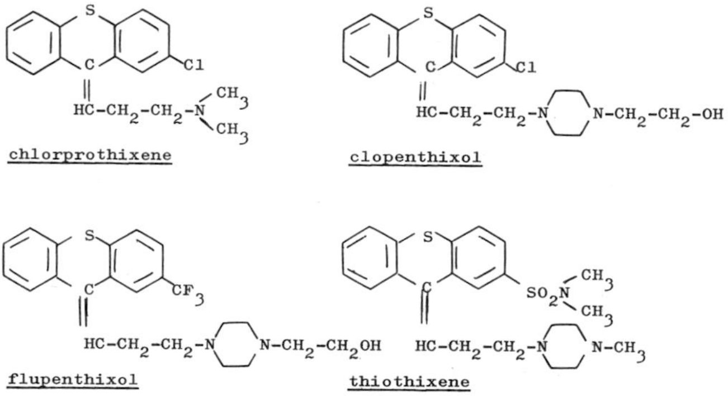

chlorprothixene clopenthixol

flupenthixol thiothixene

FIG. 4.

that they are analogs of chlorpromazine, perphenazine, fluphenazine, and thioperazine, respectively.

II. PHARMACOLOGY

Pharmacological investigation [32] of the large number of thioxanthene derivatives synthesized showed that the essential criteria for strong neuroleptic action were:

1/ Three-carbon side chain carrying a tertiary amine group.
2/ Substitution (halogen, CF_3, OCH_3 or $SO_2N(CH_3)_2$) in position 2.
3/ The double bond between carbon-9 and the side chain. When the thioxanthene nucleus is asymmetric, two isomers are formed, of which only one has strong central activity.
4/ Compounds with a 4-(hydroxyethyl)- or 4-(methyl)-piperazinylpropylidene side chain (i.e. clopenthixol, flupenthixol, and thiothixene) proved to be particularly potent neuroleptics.

Like the phenothiazines, neuroleptics of the thioxanthene series are substances with multiple pharmacological actions, both central and peripheral.[21,26,28,58] Spontaneous motor activity is reduced, chlorprothixene being slightly more potent than clopenthixol and flupenthixol. With respect to cataleptic effect, on the other hand, chlorprothixene is considerably weaker than clopenthixol, flupenthixol, and thiothixene.

Conditioned avoidance behavior is inhibited by the thioxanthenes in a specific manner. Chlorprothixene is the least potent, clopenthixol rather more so, and flupenthixol and thiothixene are the most potent with a longer-lasting effect. The antiapomorphine effect in the dog is most pronounced with thiothixene followed by flupenthixol and clopenthixol, while chlorprothixene is a rather weak antagonist. In rats, the relative antiapomorphine potencies of chlorprothixene, clopenthixol and flupenthixol have been found to be 1, 5 and 80, respectively, which corresponds well with the clinical potencies of the three drugs. On the other hand, chlorprothixene is the most powerful potentiator of anesthetics and alcohol, while flupenthixol and thiothixene are considerably weaker and clopenthixol intermediate in this respect. The temperature-lowering effect also is more pronounced with chlorprothixene than with any of the other thioxanthenes.

Peripherally, the thioxanthenes, like the phenothiazines, have α-adrenolytic properties, chlorprothixene being most potent. In the central nervous system, indirect evidence of a catecholamine-blocking effect is found in the fact that these compounds increase catecholamine turnover in the brainstem of rats (Pletscher *et al.*)[33] and in the corpus striatum of rabbits (Roos).[51]

III. DISTRIBUTION, METABOLISM AND EXCRETION [1,18,19,20,21,35]

Animal studies have shown high concentrations of the thioxanthenes in lungs, liver and kidneys. Relatively large amounts are also found in the brain, while the blood concentration is low. The thioxanthenes are extensively metabolized before excretion, only minor amounts being excreted unchanged. The main metabolic route is oxidation of ring sulfur to give sulfoxides. Besides this, dealkylation of the nitrogen in the side chain takes place to a large degree. No indication of formation of phenolic compounds has been seen. This is in contrast to the phenothiazines, where phenolic metabolites are found.

Two thioxanthenes, clopenthixol and flupenthixol, which contain an aliphatic hydroxy group in the side chain, are to a certain degree excreted as conjugation products with glucuronic acid. The thioxanthenes and their metabolites are excreted both in urine and in feces. Substances containing a piperazine group in the side chain are mainly excreted in the feces, while the excretion products of chlorprothixene are equally distributed between feces and urine.

IV. CLINICAL INTRODUCTION

Department K at Middelfart is a psychiatric state hospital department, in which are treated both newly admitted, acutely ill patients and chronic patients. It has a total of 470 beds, of which 140 are for the treatment of acutely admitted patients and 330 in the wards for chronic patients, including geriatric wards. During the past ten years, the number of admissions has varied between 800 and 1,000 patients per year. The department admits only patients suffering from neurotic or psychotic illness. Feeble-minded patients, criminal psychopaths, and epileptics are treated in Denmark in special institutions. This is a great advantage, because it provides, among other things, a better environment than that possible in departments with a more mixed clientele. We do try hard, in fact, to make the patients' surroundings in hospital as attractive as possible. We have nicely decorated walls, pleasant pictures and curtains, and furniture that matches. We are fortunate in having—compared to many other centers—a relatively large staff of attendants. We emphasize ancillary forms of therapy, such as occupational therapy, psychotherapy, social therapy, etc. With all these facilities we endeavor to establish as good a therapeutic hospital environment as possible. In addition we run follow-up and after-treatment clinics for out-patients in two towns some distance away from the hospital.

I am telling you this, not in order to boast, but because it has an important bearing on our dosage of psychopharmacological drugs. Many people have expressed surprise, in the past, at the relatively small doses that we use; this is made possible, I am sure, by the other forms of therapy, by the type of patient that we treat, and by the general therapeutic environment.

Up to 1958, we used mainly chlorpromazine, perphenazine, and reserpine in the psychopharmacological treatment of our patients, though at that time we were in the process of stopping the use of reserpine. We also used insulin coma therapy, which we discontinued in 1959, and insulin sleep, which we gave up in 1960. Lobotomy we discontinued in 1955. In addition to the pharmacological and ancillary treatments, we do, of course, use ECT; but, as a result of the increased administration of neuroleptics, and, since 1958, of antidepressant drugs, our use of this treatment is now on a very limited scale. In the period from January 1 to December 8, 1969, the department carried out 387 ECT treatments, or an average of 7.9 per week.

In 1955, we began to carry out clinical studies of psychopharmacological drugs in the department, and three years later we were introduced to the thioxanthenes.

V. CHLORPROTHIXENE (TARACTAN, TRUXAL)

The first clinical trial with chlorprothixene was initiated in the autumn of 1958. Treatment of the first patient started on November 10. On December 29, 1958, i.e., seven weeks after the trial began, we sent our first report to the firm. It contained a survey of the first 45 patients treated with chlorprothixene; 18 of them were schizophrenics. Even in this early report, dealing with comparatively few but thoroughly investigated patients, the action of chlorprothixene was clearly defined in terms that still apply after the passage of eleven years. We emphasized the sedative effect, the antipsychotic action, the antidepressant effect of small doses, and also the effect on mania and in abstinence psychoses, including psychogenic psychoses. All patients were subjected to a series of laboratory tests, and no evidence was found of nephrotoxic, hepatotoxic, or hematotoxic actions. As clinical side effects, we found drowsiness, dryness of the mouth, difficulty in accommodation, tachycardia, and increase in weight. We pointed out that we had not seen extrapyramidal symptoms.

Immediately after we had started, studies of chlorprothixene were initiated also at the Rheinische Landeskrankenhaus in Bonn, and at the Pfalzische Nervenklinik, Landeck. The experience from these departments agreed with ours [11, 24] though the numbers of patients were smaller. Subsequently, larger numbers were studied. These three clinical investigations, performed as pilot experiments, formed the total clinical evidence on the strength of which chlorprothixene was approved by the Danish Health Ministry. This approval was given on January 30, 1959, about twelve weeks after the first patient had started treatment. The drug was marketed on March 28, 1959, barely five months after the first clinical experiment.

This timing was, no doubt, too fast and, seen with today's eyes, not thorough enough. Yet has it become too difficult today to have new preparations approved? Are we not in danger of strangling at birth new preparations that, in fact, could represent a therapeutic advance? Have we not become too anxious about side effects? If Fischer and von Meering had today applied to the Danish National Health Service in respect of diemal (Veronal), it would most probably, after my investigations in the 1930's, be rejected as a specialty.[36]

The first clinical publication on chlorprothixene, a study of 70 patients, appeared in April, 1959.[23] Later I. Möller Nielsen, P. V. Petersen and I published a chemical, pharmacological and clinical survey comprising 120 patients.[29] Experience from the treatment of 258 patients was reported in 1961.[38] The first controlled experiment was carried out at the beginning of 1959,[37] in which chlorprothixene proved superior to placebo. This was later confirmed by, among others, Scanlan and May.[52] In a controlled comparison of chlorprothixene and chlorpromazine, Remvig and Sonne[48] found chlorprothixene to be the better drug on account, inter alia, of its lower toxicity. Cappelen and Monrad came to a similar conclusion.[6] Arnold[2] and also Gross[14] describe chlorprothixene as a broad-spectrum neuroleptic with few and harmless side effects. There is, however, insufficient time to deal fully with the voluminous literature on the subject. The antidepressant effect of chlorprothixene has been the subject of much discussion, but seems now to have been established by Kielholz,[22] among others.

We have almost completely gone over, particularly in the chronic wards, to treating our patients with thioxanthenes. On December 1, 1969, one patient in these wards was receiving chlorpromazine and six perphenazine, while the rest were treated with thioxanthenes. As shown in Table 5, we have treated a very large number of patients with chlorprothixene, either alone or in combination with other forms of therapy and other psychopharmacological drugs.

If I were to summarize why we are so satisfied with chlorpro-

TABLE 5.

Total to 1st November, 1969:	
Chlorprothixene alone	4,438 patients
Chlorprothixene in combinations	3,663
total:	8,101 patients

thixene, my answer would be that it is a broad-spectrum neuroleptic with very few, and rarely troublesome, side effects. In particular, there are practically no extrapyramidal symptoms; there are no toxic effects on bone marrow or liver; and no contact dermatitis or photosensitization, either. Chlorprothixene is effective in a variety of psychotic conditions; it is easy to use for children and as supportive therapy in neuroses. It is highly effective in genuine, severe migraine, and in several other conditions, which there is not time to touch on here.

VI. CLOPENTHIXOL (CIATYL, SORDINOL)

In 1959, we added perphenazine to the treatment of some patients who were not responding adequately to chlorprothixene, and obtained good results from this combination. At a research meeting with Messrs. H. Lundbeck & Co., it turned out that the firm had made an analogue of perphenazine in the thioxanthene series. This analogue, clopenthixol, was, therefore examined more closely by experiments on animals. After that we carried out the initial clinical investigations at Middelfart, where the first patient was given the drug on November 7, 1959, almost exactly one year after the first thioxanthene derivative had been clinically tested.

Even by that time, things did not proceed fast. On January 28, 1960, we submitted a preliminary report, and on October 10, 1960, after almost one year had elapsed, we followed this with a final report dealing with 40 patients. We concluded that, in a study lasting for several months, we had found clopenthixol to have a good sedative effect with a powerful antipsychotic action, more marked than that of chlorpromazine and similar to that of perphenazine. Extrapyramidal symptoms were seen during treatment with clopenthixol, but they seemed less severe than those produced by perphenazine, and were easy to control by antiparkinson agents. Among other side actions, we observed tachycardia in 15% of the patients, and in 41% a slight fall in blood pressure, which in only two was of orthostatic type. The remaining side effects were quite mild. Laboratory tests showed no evidence of liver damage and no hematotoxic or nephrotoxic action. We pointed out that we were using moderate doses, and yet we observed good effects.

After further evaluation in other clinics, clopenthixol was marketed on December 2, 1961. This time, therefore, it took two years, and not, as with chlorprothixene, less than half a year. The first publication comprised 97 patients [39, 40]; among them were 56 schizophrenics, of whom only four remained unaffected by the treatment and one became worse. In addition, small groups of patients with other diagnoses were treated; these included 14 patients with severe forms of neuroses, where a clear anxiety-reducing effect was observed. It was suggested that clopenthixol might be of value in geriatrics administered, however, in very small doses. This was confirmed later by Dahl [7] and also by Malmgren and Ohnell.[25]

In 1964, a paper was published reporting 252 patients; 112 were schizophrenics,[41] and in them a useful effect was observed in 80%. This was confirmed by Sourander and Kaartinen,[55] who carried out a double-blind comparative study between chlorpromazine and clopenthixol, which came out in favor of clopenthixol. The authors stress (as we ourselves do) that one should use low dosages. Hildebrand [17] treated 298 psychotic patients and claimed a percentage improvement rate of 92; among his patients were 198 schizophrenics. Ban and his colleagues [3] state that clopenthixol is especially suitable for the treatment of chronic schizophrenic patients who are otherwise resistant to treatment. Bartolucci and his colleagues [4] have shown in a controlled experiment that in the treatment of chronic patients, clopenthixol is as effective as perphenazine, and better than chlorprothixene. In 1965, we examined at Middelfart all patients in the chronic wards under the age of 70, who had been taking psychopharmacological drugs for more than five years. The total came to 191 patients. Only 3 of them or 1.5% showed excitomotor phenomena, 1 on clopenthixol, and 2 on perphenazine. The phenomena vanished completely when treatment was changed to chlorprothixene. The proportion of patients with extrapyramidal symptoms is shown in Table 6.

This agrees well with Sourander and Kaartinen [55] who found that 35% of patients showed extrapyramidal symptoms during treatment with clopenthixol.

TABLE 6.

	CHLORPROTHIXENE	CLOPENTHIXOL	CLOPENTHIXOL + CHLORPROTHIXENE	PERPHENAZINE
No. of patients	48	69	41	18
Extrapyramidal symptoms in %	0	39	32	78

Our practice is now as a matter of routine always to give an antiparkinson drug when we treat a patient with clopenthixol, and we very seldom observe side effects. In addition, we increasingly use combined treatment with chlorprothixene and clopenthixol, giving a small dose of clopenthixol in the evening. During recent years we have also combined methylperidol (Luvatrena) and clopenthixol, again giving the latter substance in the evening.[45] In Table 7 a survey is given of the number of patients treated with clopenthixol alone and in combination with other preparations.

TABLE 7.

Total to 1st November, 1969:	
Clopenthixol alone	2,347 patients
Clopenthixol in combinations	1,705
total:	4,052 patients

Last year, we subjected 57 patients, who have been treated with clopenthixol alone over a period from three to nine years, to a long series of laboratory tests. Rud and I[47] found no evidence of any hematotoxic, hepatotoxic, or nephrotoxic effects. Electrocardiograms and measurements of blood pressure carried out by the orthostatic method also showed nothing abnormal.

To summarize clopenthixol, we feel we can say that here is another thioxanthene derivative that seems to show fewer side effects than other similar neuroleptics and a clinical effect that is just as good, if not better.

VII. FLUPENTHIXOL (FLUANXOL)

The first clinical studies of flupenthixol were carried out by Gross and Kaltenbäck in Vienna,[15] who started their work in May, 1963. In their publication, the authors describe their results in 570 patients, 90% of whom were schizophrenics. They conclude that flupenthixol is a neuroleptic of medium therapeutic action. It is neither a basal neuroleptic like chlorprothixene, nor as intense in its action as clopenthixol. Only 4% of the patients showed sedation, thus the preparation is suitable for the treatment of quiet schizophrenics, in whom the antipsychotic effect is excellent. The authors used antiparkinson agents routinely but nevertheless had to discontinue flupenthixol in 22 patients on account of severe extrapyramidal disturbances. Other side effects, which were not serious, were found in 27% of the patients. Põldinger[34] has compared 100 patients treated with chlorprothixene with 100 treated with clopenthixol and 50 treated with flupenthixol. The first two drugs had a good sedative and antipsychotic effect, while flupenthixol had mainly an antipsychotic effect, acting almost specifically on delusions, hallucinations and thought disorder.

We started our clinical investigations at Middelfart on November 16, 1963; it seems that we have a strong preference for starting our experiments in the month of November. We studied flupenthixol as an adjuvant in the treatment of neuroses,[42] 34 patients taking part in our pilot experiment. We found that the preparation had an exceptionally good anxiety-reducing effect and a rapid onset of action. We saw some evidence of extrapyramidal symptoms, but apart from that there were very few side effects. Flupenthixol was approved by the Danish Health Department on November 15, 1965, and was marketed in January, 1966. Sonne has stated that flupenthixol, given in small doses, has a good effect on patients with endogenous depressions.[54] However, we observed the antidepressant effect particularly in patients with atypical depressions.[43]

We have also used flupenthixol at Middelfart in the treatment of quiet schizophrenic patients, in neuroses, and in ambulatory aftercare, where it is a big advantage that the drug has no sedative action. Table 8 shows how many patients we have treated with flupenthixol, alone or in combination, up to November 1, 1969:

TABLE 8.

Total to 1st November, 1969:	
Flupenthixol alone	367 patients
Flupenthixol in combinations	158
total:	525 patients

Of the combinations, I wish to emphasize the use of flupenthixol plus clopenthixol in the treatment of schizophrenics, who are given flupenthixol in the daytime and clopenthixol at night.

We have also combined flupenthixol with melitracene (Dixeran, Thymeol, trausabun), first in free combination, and in the last two years as a trial preparation with a fixed dose-ratio. The combination has been used in the treatment of neuroses, and we have observed good antidepressant and anxiolytic effects. The combination of a neuroleptic and a thymoleptic leads to a reduced or negligible incidence of extrapyramidal symptoms. Altogether, we have treated 70 patients with this combination.[46] Gottfries repeating a controlled trial comparing flupenthixol and trifluoperazine, found the preparations to be equally effective. In both groups approximately 30% of the patients showed extrapyramidal symptoms.[13]

The latest form of therapy with flupenthixol is to give the substance in depot form, administered by injection every second to every fourth week. Remvig and his colleagues[49] emphasize that chronic, quiet schizophrenics especially show considerable improvement. Fatigue decreases, autism and negativism diminish, and mood improves. Extrapyramidal symptoms occurred fairly frequently, but were easily controlled by antiparkinson drugs. These observations have been confirmed by Rimestad,[50] Gjestland,[12] and Enerheim *et al.*,[9] who studied as many as 99 patients. Stucke[56] treated 256 patients with similarly good results; his series included 53 patients with endogenous depressions who apparently also showed a satisfactory response. His experience in the treatment of schizophrenics agrees with what we have seen so far in Middelfart.

Summarizing the results with flupenthixol, I can say that the substance has a good antipsychotic effect; it has no sedative action and is, therefore, particularly suitable for ambulatory after-treatment. And I shouldn't wonder if the depot type of preparation was the treatment of the future.

VIII. THIOTHIXENE (NAVANE)

Finally, I shall mention the latest thioxanthene derivative, thiothixene, which is the thioxanthene analogue of thioproperazine (Majeptil). I have no personal experience with the preparation, which was synthesized by Pfizer & Co. in Connecticut, USA, in 1965.

Sugermann *et al.*,[57] in an uncontrolled trial, found moderate improvement in 50% of chronic schizophrenic patients, while Gann[10] reports a good effect in 66%. In a controlled study, Paquay[30] found that the preparation was a potent and reliable neuroleptic having an action similar to that of large doses of chlorpromazine. Haase *et al.*,[16] in an uncontrolled trial, observed a very good effect in 40% of patients suffering from acute schizophrenia, while Bishop *et al.*[5] found under controlled conditions that the action of thiothixene was equal to that of trifluoperazine. Wolpert *et al.*[59] consider thiothixene to be slightly more effective than thioridazine. Skovgaard Jensen and his colleagues[53] report a pilot study in 34 schizophrenics, 65% of whom showed a moderate to good response. The side effects seem, in contrast to those reported with thioproperazine, to be relatively mild and mainly of extrapyramidal nature.

In conclusion, I should like to state that in Department K at Middelfart, we have proved for several years that one can generally manage with a therapeutic armamentarium consisting of the existing thioxanthenes, particularly in the treatment of chronic patients. I believe that the patients feel better with these substances and I prefer them to the phenothiazines, in particular, chlorpromazine. In the treatment of chronic patients, I think they are to be preferred to the butyrophenones, because the thioxanthenes do not cause such severe extrapyramidal symptoms as the butyrophenones do.

My final words in this chapter should be, and are, my sincere thanks to my friends the chemist, P. V. Petersen, and the pharmacologist, I. Möller Nielsen, for their invaluable collaboration over many years.

REFERENCES

1. Allgen, L-G., *et al.:* Experimentia *16:*325, 1960.
2. Arnold, O. H.: Wien Med Wschr *109:*892, 1959.
3. Ban, T. A., *et al.:* Amer J Psychiat *119:*984, 1963.
4. Bartolucci, G., *et al.:* Curr Ther Res *8:*581, 1966.
5. Bishop, M. P., *et al.: Ibid.*, p. 509.
6. Cappelen, T., and Monrad, H.: T Norsk Laegeforen *81:*486, 1961.
7. Dahl, R.: Ugeskr Laeg *127:*712, 1965.
8. Dunitz, J. D., *et al.:* Helv Chim Acta *47:*1897, 1964.
9. Enerheim, B., *et al.:* Nord Psykiat T, 1970, in press.
10. Gann, G.: Wien Med Wschr *118:*10, 1968.
11. Geller, W.: Med Klin *55:*554, 1960.
12. Gjestland, A.: T Norsk Laegeforen, 1970, in press.
13. Gottfries, C-G.: In press.
14. Gross, H.: Wien Med Wschr *110:*718, 1960.
15. Gross, H., and Kaltenbäck, E.: Acta Psychiat Scan *41:*42, 1965.
16. Haase, H., *et al.:* Arzneimittelforschung *17:*1043, 1967.
17. Hildebrand, H-J.: Deutsch Med J *15:*242, 1964.
18. Hobbs, D. C.: J Pharm Sci *57:*105, 1968.
19. Huus, I., and Rauf Khan, A.: Acta Pharmacol (Kobenhavn) *25:*397, 1967.
20. Jörgensen, A., *et al.: Ibid.* *27:*301, 1969.
21. Khan, F. Rauf: *Ibid.*, p. 202.
22. Kielholz, P.: Psychiatrische Pharmakotherapie in Klinik and Praxis, Bern und Stuttgart, 1965.
23. Madsen, E., and Ravn, J.: Nord Psykiat T *8:*82, 1959.
24. Mall, G.: Symposium at Cologne, June 6, 1959.
25. Malmgren, G., and Ohnell, L. K.: Svensk Läkartidn *60:*1630, 1963.
26. Möller Nielsen, I.: Nord Psykiat T *21:*424, 1967.
27. ——: Mod Probl Pharmacopsychiat *2:*23, 1969.
28. Möller Nielsen, I., and Neuhold, K.: Acta Pharmacol (Kobenhavn) *15:* 335, 1959.

29. Möller Nielsen, I., Petersen, P. V., and Ravn, J.: Ugeskr Laeg *121*:1433, 1959.
30. Paquay, J., *et al.*: Belgian Society of Mental Medicine, Juni, 1968.
31. Petersen, P. V., *et al.*: Arzneimittelforschung *8*:395, 1958.
32. Petersen, P. V., and Müller Nielsen, I.: Psychopharmacological Agents, vol. 1, New York, Acad Press, 1964, p. 301.
33. Pletscher, A., *et al.*: Proc Europ Soc Drug Toxicity *9*:98, 1968.
34. Pöldinger, W.: Arzneimittelforschung *17*:1133, 1967.
35. Raaflaub, J.: *Ibid.*, p. 1391.
36. Ravn, J:. Om visse fejlkilder ved haematologiske undersegelser af skizofrene, (with English summary). Disp. Copenhagen, 1950.
37. ——: Wien Klin Wschr 72:192, 1960.
38. ——: Amer J Psychiat *118*:227, 1961.
39. Ravn, J., and Rud, C.: Ugeskr Laeg *123*:1663, 1961.
40. Ravn, J.: Med Klin *57*:1227, 1962.
41. Ravn, J.: *et al.*: Neuropsychopharmacology *3*:286, 1964.
42. Ravn, J., and Rud, C.: Nord Psykiat T *19*:66, 1965.
43. Ravn, J.: *Ibid. 20*:410, 1966.
44. ——: *Ibid. 21*:401, 1967.
45. ——: *Ibid. 23*:13, 1969.
46. ——: *Ibid.*, 1970, in press.
47. Ravn, J., and Rud, C.: In press.
48. Remvig, J., and Sonne, L. M.: Psychopharmacotherapia *2*:203, 1961.
49. Remvig, J., *et al.*: Nord Psykiat T *22*:392, 1968.
50. Rimestad, S.: Personal communication.
51. Roos, B-E.: J Pharm Pharmacol *17*:820, 1965.
52. Scanlan, E. P., and May, A. E.: Brit J Psychiat *109*:418, 1963.
53. Skovgaard Jensen, P., *et al.*: Nord Psykiat T *23*:(#4), 1969.
54. Sonne, L. M.: *Ibid. 20*:322, 1966.
55. Sourander, C., and Kaartinen, M.: *Ibid. 17*:83, 1963.
56. Stucke, W.: Das ärztliche Gespräch, Symposium at Cologne, November 14, 1969.
57. Sugermann, A. A., *et al.*: Curr Ther Res 7:810, 1965.
58. Weissman, A.: Mod Probl Pharmacopsychiat *2*:15, 1969.
59. Wolpert, A., *et al.*: Curr Ther Res *9*:482, 1967.

CHAPTER

15

Monoamine Oxidase Inhibitors: An Unfinished Picaresque Tale

NATHAN S. KLINE, MD, FACP *

"His vital force of mind, a conqueror
Beyond the flaming ramparts of the world"
Lucretius: *De Rerum Natura*

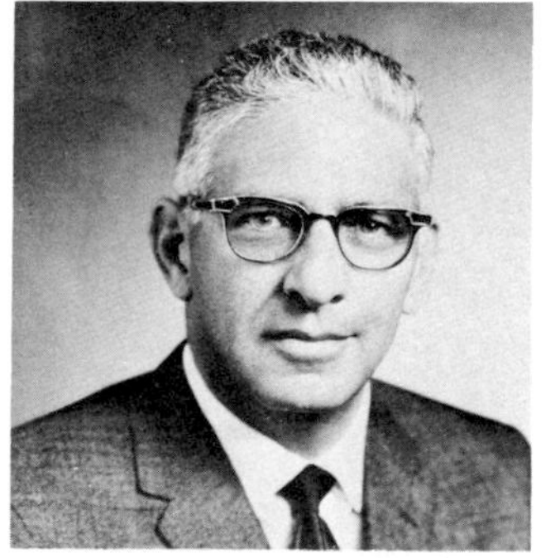

RESEARCH SCIENTISTS are wide-eyed manipulators. When an observant brat discovers for the first time that he can push buttons, turn faucets, open doors, dial phone numbers and exploit his parents, he is astonished and delighted at this ability to uncover and control the physical and social environment. Some of us never recover.

Until fairly recent times, the researcher was paid substantially less than those earning an honest living. In many cases this was because he felt guilty taking *any* money at all for doing something he so much enjoyed. This position is not quite so ridiculous as it sounds since the Royal Society in England was formed by wealthy gentlemen for the sheer pleasure of carrying out experiments. We are not only granted these extraordinary prerogatives, but equipment and supplies are provided to us plus a salary to boot.

Few joys equal the realization of fantasies in which a successful

* Director, Research Center, Rockland State Hospital, Orangeburg, New York; Director, Psychiatric Services, Bergen Pines County Hospital, Paramus, New Jersey; Associate Clinical Professor of Psychiatry, Columbia University College of Psysicians and Surgeons, New York; psychiatric practice, New York.

researcher indulges or, for that matter, few joys equal the fantasies themselves. Imagine being able to spend a whole lifetime just poking around to see what will happen. The fact that the questioning and answering is sophisticated and according to certain rules doesn't change the basic activity. For those of a mechanical bent it is possible not only to keep on purchasing the most intriguing Erector Sets but sometimes even to have one built to specifications.

If you like to sleep late and work in the evening, no one really objects and, if the work gets a bit dull, it's always justified to visit a laboratory (located in some seasonal climate) that is doing the same sort of activity. If you climb high enough up the hierarchy, you can then direct others to carry out all sorts of interesting things that you don't have time to do yourself. One of the sweetest smells in the world, that of fresh galley proofs, is an added attraction; the absolute power to add to, subtract from, and alter an article that is to become part of the world's "permanent" literature guarantees temporary immortality.

The apogee of the whole voyage occurs when something New reveals itself to you (whether it later proves to be incorrect or not is irrelevant). You have found a missing piece in the jigsaw puzzle! You have forged a passkey which might open innumerable closed doors! I will never forget the picture of Linus Pauling in a meeting at McGill describing the creative process. He rubbed his hands in pure sensual satisfaction and his baby-blue eyes positively glittered: "Just think," he said, "I know something that no one else in the whole wide world knows—and they won't know it until I tell them."

A hundred years from now our names will be impersonally listed in a book or in the memory bank of a computer or perhaps erased completely. Yet medicine and science will be Just That Much Different because we have lived; treatment and understanding of illness will forever be altered even though the alteration is no longer perceptible, and in our own way we will persist for all time in that small contribution we have made toward the Human Venture.

"History is but the lengthened shadow of a man" *Emerson*

In the spring of 1953, we needed funds to purchase a Scholander apparatus for some gas analyses. Arthur Dale Console was then

Medical Director of Squibb, and we saw each other on occasion socially. When I asked whether Squibb could make us a grant for the amount needed, he indicated that drug house support was given either for product development or for goodwill—and no pharmaceutical company really cared whether or not it was well thought of by those in psychiatric hospitals since the only drugs sold were some sedatives and a small amount of insulin. We therefore scratched around to find some potential new product, and finally came up with *Rauwolfia serpentina* (only 2,000 years old!). Vakil reporting in a British journal, and subsequently Wilkins in Boston, much to everyone's surprise, had found rauwolfia useful in reducing hypertension just as the Ayurvedic literature claimed. Since the drug was also advocated for snake bite, toxemia of pregnancy, insanity and half a dozen other disorders, we put in a request for $1,000 to evaluate rauwolfia in psychiatric patients. While we were setting up the study, it was announced that Ciba had isolated one of the rauwolfia alkaloids, reserpine. With a number of our staff, we went to Summit to see if we could persuade them to allow us to compare not only Rauwolfia and placebo but Rauwolfia, reserpine and placebo. This netted us a few thousand more dollars toward our basic research and we undertook a study of 710 patients. The study was completed late in 1953 and presented under the auspices of the New York Academy of Sciences on February 5, 1954.

The almost simultaneous introduction of chlorpromazine added great impetus to the beginnings of the psychopharmacological revolution. Two years later I gave my one and only address to the American Psychoanalytic Association. The senior author was Mortimer Ostow, and we had spent the better part of a year on and off discussing the possible mode of action of reserpine and chlorpromazine in everything from neurophysiological to psychoanalytic terms. Utilizing both general systems approach and the classic psychoanalytic doctrine in which the universe is divided into psychotopology (id, ego, superego), psychodynamics, and psychoenergetics, we not only "explained" the action of reserpine and chlorpromazine but also postulated the existence of drugs that would function as antidepressants (or *psychic energizers,* as I subsequently designated them). Let me read you what we had to say in 1956 under the heading of "Validation."

We have here presented a hypothesis concerning the nature of the action of reserpine and chlorpromazine. We have constructed the hypothesis in such a way as to account for all the data that have come to our attention. We can offer no more convincing proof that our hypothesis is correct. In this paper the only supporting evidence we can propose is the capacity of the hypothesis to unify all the known facts. If it can do that, it has a certain value. Its validity will ultimately be determined by whether it can lead us to new information and useful understanding.

For example, one may ask, "What would be the clinical properties of a drug which facilitated the generation of psychic energy, if such a drug could be found?" Our hypotheses would lead us to the following predictions. It would relieve simple depression and at least the sadness and inertia of melancholia when aggression is present. It would reduce the sleep requirement and delay the onset of fatigue. It would increase appetite and sexual desire and increase behavioral drive in general. Motor and intellectual activity would be speeded up. It would heighten responsiveness to stimuli, both pleasant and noxious, not by improving the function of apperception, but by increasing the readiness to respond to percepts that release instinctual behavior. The plethora of id energy would make large amounts of energy easily available to the ego so that there would be more than enough energy available for all tasks. Such a situation would result in a sense of a joyousness and optimism. As the dose was raised to the point where id drives threatened the integrity of the ego, anxiety would appear. If the dose was raised still further, one would expect the id pressure finally to cause a rupture of ego defenses so that clinical neurosis or psychosis would ensue, depending upon the specific ego weakness which would determine its line of fracture. Such a drug might be helpful for the management of inertia and depression in parkinsonism.

In May, 1956, we received a visit from Dr. Severinghaus, Medical Director of Hoffmann-LaRoche, who was also searching for an antidepressant drug. He was properly much impressed with the antidepressant action of opiates and had been working on the possibility of developing a nonaddicting opiate with such antidepressant action.

On April 11, 1956, I had lectured at the Warner Laboratories in Morris Plains, New Jersey. Afterwards I visited Dr. Charles Scott, who was just completing researches that he felt would be of particular interest to me in view of the role I had played in the introduction of reserpine. Dr. Chessin and he had found that if experimental animals were given iproniazid prior to reserpine that instead of becoming calm and somewhat sedated they actually became hyperalert and hyperactive. The possibility of using this combination on retarded and depressed patients immediately led me to speculate whether this was the psychic energizer for which we had all been looking. I mentioned the possibility to Dr. S. Evert Svenson of Hoffmann-LaRoche, with whom I was in contact because of early testing on one of the precursors of Librium. He told me to raise the possibility when Dr. Severinghaus visited us. Notification was sent to the FDA. Dr. Severinghaus at the time of his visit on May 19, 1956, was singularly *unimpressed* with the idea, although he did confirm the fact that Dr. Pletscher, the Research Director of Hoffmann-LaRoche in Switzerland, working with Dr. B. B. Brodie and P. Shore at the National Institutes of Health in Washington, had independently carried out the same investigations as had Scott and Chessin and gotten the same results. For all practical purposes, the use of iproniazid in treating tuberculosis had been replaced by isoniazid, which had many fewer side effects. Were it not for a few clinicians such as Bosworth, who insisted that iproniazid was superior for tuberculosis of the bone, Roche would have discontinued sale of the drug entirely.

John Saunders had joined our staff May 24 of that same year, having previously worked with Ciba, where his job was to help stimulate and collaborate with clinical investigators in the field. When I described the animal experiments, he was quite interested in possible applications of iproniazid for a number of pharmacological reasons. This was listed as one of the projects to be under his supervision and I proceeded to obtain reprints of prior publications on iproniazid from the New York Academy of Medicine. Much to my surprise, I found reports that psychiatric patients had already been treated. Jackson Smith at Baylor University was in a neighboring lab to Vernon John Kinross-Wright, who in 1953 was working on the tranquilizing action of chlorpromazine. In August of 1953, Smith reported on results of 11 patients treated for a period of two to three weeks. Unfortunately, he was evaluating iproniazid as a *tranquilizer*. Despite the relatively short time, he did note that two of the depressed patients showed some improvement, but all in all concluded that the drug was ineffectual as a tranquilizer. That same year Kamman *et al.* reported the effect on chronic psychiatric patients in a double-blind study and found definite improvement in ward behavior of 30 patients tested. The authors concluded that although the medication was definitely superior to placebo used in a comparable group of 30 patients, it was not as effective as a "total push program" in a third group of 30 patients. Hence it was dropped from investigation. Other data on the side effects described euphoria and elation in patients treated for tuberculosis, but this had inspired no one with thoughts that it might be an antidepressant.

There were undoubtedly several others who worked with iproniazid even earlier than Smith, Kamman and ourselves but who did not report their results. Interestingly enough, among these was Dr. Ayd, who had begun such clinical trials as early as 1952 or 1953. All in all, he gave the medication to several hundred patients but, possibly because the drug takes so long to work, did not notice any consistent improvement. Based on the report of our own findings, he reexamined his past cases and started clinical trials once again.

In an effort to elicit cooperation from non-Research Center staff members at Rockland State Hospital, we had adopted the policy of making them senior authors of any studies in which they collaborated. Dr. Harry Loomer was temporarily placed in charge of a group of patients when one of the senior physicians went on vacation. At lunch one day, he asked Dr. Saunders whether we at Research had any treatment for retarded and regressed patients who had failed to respond to reserpine and/or chlorpromazine. This was precisely the type of collaboration for which we were seeking, and Dr. Saunders arranged with Dr. Loomer to carry out the investigation we had planned.

During the first few days in November, 1956, 17 hospital patients were started on iproniazid. The situation was somewhat complicated by the fact that a number of the patients were already on reserpine. At that time we did not know whether the behavior of the experimental animals was due to the combination of reserpine and iproniazid, to iproniazid followed by reserpine, or to iproniazid alone. Of course, we also did not know whether patients would react the same way as the experimental animals. Hence for the majority of the patients involved in the study we discontinued all medications except iproniazid. The official diagnoses on the hospital patients was dementia praecox. At the same time I began looking for suitable patients with *depression* in my private practice and also discussed possible treatment along these lines with two colleagues, Dr. Samuel Sandler and Dr. Herbert Spiegel. Treatment of these patients seen in private practice was started in January of 1957, a few months after the hospital work had begun.

By February, it was obvious to us that we were really on to something exciting. There were reasonably frequent visits from Dr. S. Evert Svenson of Hoffmann-LaRoche, who became caught up in our enthusiasm, but had great difficulty in trying to convince Dr. Severinghaus that Roche should pursue more extensive investigations of the drug even though it had been discovered by Dr. Fox in the Nutley, New Jersey, laboratories of the company. Here indeed was a fairly unique situation! A group of clinical investigators were trying to convince a pharmaceutical house that they had a valuable product rather than the other way around. Dr. Severinghaus remained adamantly skeptical and eventually we arranged a clandestine conference with Mr. L. David Barney, the president of the company, who received us "secretly" at Theodore's Restaurant in New York for lunch. In the flush of excellent food and wine, we were able at least to bring the matter to attention.

By happy coincidence, at that time I was Chairman of the Committee on Research of the American Psychiatric Association and two years earlier had, with the help of Mr. Robert Robinson of the American Psychiatric Association, been able to convince Ciba to underwrite the cost of publishing the Regional Research Conferences sponsored by our Committee on Research.

As Chairman of the Committee on Research, I was well informed about the Conferences and was usually asked to participate. At this point, Dr. Svenson showed me a paper submitted for publication by Dr. George Crane, in which he made reference to the success of iproniazid in the treatment of chronically fatigued tuberculosis patients with a variety of psychiatric disorders. We made the decision that even though the total number of our cases was small, since the Regional Research Conference to be held at Syracuse in April, 1957, was "Research on Affects," the work should be presented there. At the time of the meeting, we had data on only 17 regressed and retarded hospital patients and nine depressed patients seen in private practice on an ambulatory basis. Last-minute changes were made to accommodate our paper, but there was no time to add to the program the work of Dr. Crane, which had come along even later, so that he was included as a discussant of our paper, although it was for the purpose of allowing him to present his own results.

There was then another "show-down" meeting with the group from Hoffmann-LaRoche, at which time we announced that we intended to present the paper regardless of whether the company would supply further quantities of the drug or sponsor research in its application to psychiatry. At the penultimate moment, since we were going ahead in any case, the company made the decision to support our efforts.

Dr. Saunders and I had reviewed the data submitted by Dr. Loomer, and we went through several prolonged sessions with the dictaphone in my office to get together a presentable paper in time for the meeting. Problems began almost at once, since we had to persuade Dr. Loomer to dispense with an entirely inappropriate introduction that he had written. A few days before the paper was presented at Syracuse, a press conference was held in New York, at which Dr. Herbert Spiegel, in addition to ourselves, discussed some of the results. When the paper was given on Saturday afternoon, April 6, we accorded the honor of reading it to Dr. Loomer in furtherance of the policy of encouraging collaboration with the regular hospital staff. Unfortunately, the *New York Times* reported that it was I who had made the presentation, which was largely the case in respect to the press conference. This was the first paper of which Dr. Loomer was an author or coauthor and his reaction to being overlooked was a sizable one. As requested, the *New York Times* printed a retraction, indicating that it was Dr. Loomer who had read the paper.

As is often the case, it was a full year later until the proceedings of the conference were published. Due to another happy set of circumstances, however, the paper was included in my testimony before the Subcommittee of the Committee on Appropriations of the United States Senate, Eighty-fifth Congress, on May 9, 1957, a month after the presentation at Syracuse. There are some interesting differences between the manuscript as given in Syracuse and before the Congressional Committee as contrasted with the final publication. The section dealing with "theoretical considerations" was added subsequent to the original presentation. References also were made in the original paper to the investigations then under way to determine whether iproniazid followed by reserpine was more effective than iproniazid alone. On page 1385, the testimony reads: "The original plan of investigation, based on the animal experiments, called for the "pretreatment" of patients with iproniazid, which was to be followed by the administration of reserpine. It was obviously first necessary to determine the effect of iproniazid alone, since if reserpine were added before the effects of the first drug could be evaluated, it would be impossible to determine whether any beneficial results were due to the iproniazid or to the combination of the iproniazid and reserpine. Another group of patients of a similar type are being treated by relatively brief induction courses of iproniazid, followed within a week by the addition of reserpine." In June of 1957, we presented some of the data on the patients given iproniazid followed by reserpine. The results did not appear to be materially better than iproniazid used alone.

In the meantime, a fairly heated discussion had developed among workers in the field whether the antidepressant action of iproniazid was due to the fact that it was a hydrazine derivative (also used in rocket fuel at the time) or because it was a monoamine oxidase inhibitor. In the original paper at Syracuse, part of Dr. Saunder's contribution had been the attribution of the mode of action to the monoamine oxidase activity. He was subsequently vindicated when a number of nonhydrazine monoamine oxidase inhibitors were also shown to be active. Obviously there are other factors at work, since some of the most potent MAO inhibitors in the laboratory have weak or absent antidepressant activity in vivo.

Probably no drug in history was so widely used so soon after announcement of its application in the treatment of a specific disease. This circumstance arose not only because of overwhelming need for an effective antidepressant medication but also because the drug was already on the market, albeit for the treatment of tuberculosis. During the first year following our paper, there was close agreement between the pharmaceutical company and the Food and Drug Administration how many patients were treated—approximately 400,000. Oscar Wilde once said "Nothing succeeds like excess," but in this case there was an unfortunate "side effect" of the widespread usage. Some of the patients on iproniazid developed fractures of the femur while skiing. Some of the males became balder than they were before, and some patients developed jaundice. The germane question, of course, was whether any of these changes were due to iproniazid. It was only the cases of jaundice that were reported in the literature and, considering that 400,000 patients were treated, it might have been anticipated that a least 100 would have developed jaundice even though they were not on medication. The FDA, usually so insistent upon control groups, sometimes tends to forget about them when it comes to potential side effects. There actually were 127 cases of jaundice reported. However, if one stratifies the patients in respect to age and sex, it is evident that such groups as postmenopausal females are more prone to the disorder and tend to have a rougher course than younger females. Based on a review of the admittedly inadequate literature of incidence of jaundice in the general population, it appeared on the basis of the number of cases reported that iproniazid might be a good drug to use in order to *prevent* jaundice. Since there were no controls, iproniazid was immediately implicated as the causative agent. Unfortunately, studies of antibody titers in relatives of these patients were never done, so that the question of whether these were really cases of viral hepatitis or drug-induced reactions has never been settled. Hoffmann-LaRoche in the meantime had been working on other monoamine oxidase inhibitors and had come on one which, based on biochemical testing in the laboratory, was infinitely superior to iproniazid (Marsilid). Hence, as soon as any question was raised about Marsilid, they voluntarily withdrew it from the market and pushed investigation and sales of Marplan. As happens all so frequently, Marplan was vastly *inferior* to Marsilid. Other countries that did not act so precipitously still produce and sell Marsilid, with the result that there is a small but persistent black market in the drug for patients who fail to respond to other antidepressants.

Actually, there are only four patients legally on Marsilid in the entire United States. One is a patient of mine who did extremely well on the medication—even giving birth to her second child, having been on the drug all through pregnancy up to the time of delivery. Just at the time of the birth, the drug was withdrawn from the market and she was placed on an identical-appearing placebo. She promptly went downhill and the substitution of other antidepressant drugs was totally inadequate. Finally, in desperation, she wrote to the FDA with "before-and-after" photographs. I was granted an exemption to reinstitute the treatment in her case. She immediately responded and has remained on the drug for the past five or six years. From time to time, Hoffmann-LaRoche produces a new batch of Marsilid in part to keep my one patient happy.

Later events include other MAO inhibitors; the pressure of the medical profession to have Parnate remarketed after the FDA had removed it; contention who had contributed what in the original psychiatric usage; discovery of the role of tyramine in producing side effects at certain times and in certain patients; and the combination of MAO inhibitors with tricyclic antidepressants as the most potent treatment for otherwise drug-resistant depressed patients.

Locked in the monoamine oxidase inhibitor story is not only the secret of treating depression but the key to its cause and prevention. This door is beginning to open, and behind it we find even now evidence that the mechanisms of schizophrenia and perhaps even some of the neuroses will become visible and treatable. I began with a quotation from Lucretius, let me close with another from his contemporary, Virgil:

> "Audacibus annue coeptis"—
> "Happy is he who learns the causes of things".

CHAPTER 16

The Imipramine Story

ROLAND KUHN, MD *

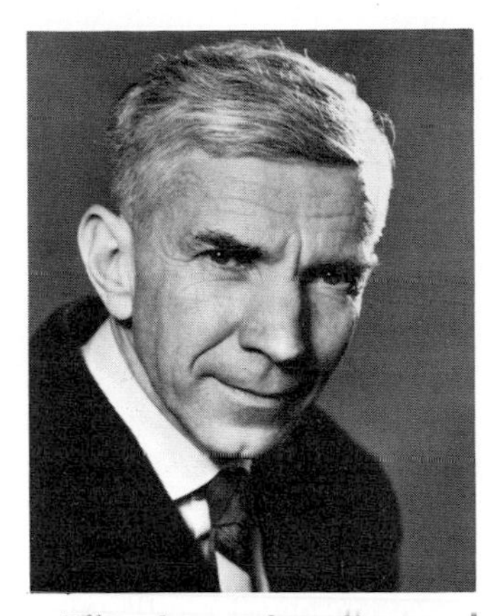

THE IMIPRAMINE STORY can be divided into its previous history, the story of its discovery, and the further history of this antidepressant drug since the first publication of September 1957. The discovery of imipramine as an antidepressive agent has its roots in the whole history of the depressive diseases. But it is closely tied also to the discoverer's own life story.

HISTORICAL

The depressive diseases involve much suffering for not only the patient but also his family. They are dangerous and very widespread. Their study has always appealed to the inquisitive mind of man, particularly of course that of the doctor. Our knowledge of the history of depression—known earlier as *melancholy*—has been much extended in all directions during the last few years. Thus Flashar has written on *Melancholy and the Melancholic in the Medical Theories of the Ancients*, Klibansky, Saxl and Panofsky have gathered together the concepts of the Middle Ages under the title *Saturn and Melancholy*, and Wyrsch has thrown fresh light on scientific ideas about manic-depressive psychosis during the last hundred years in an unusually wide-ranging survey. Finally, we are indebted to Starobinski for his *History of the Treatment of Melancholy from the Earliest Times until 1900.*

The modern discovery that depression can be treated by drugs

* The Cantonal Psychiatric Clinic, Münsterlingen, Switzerland—Director: Dr. A. Zolliker.

originated in the basic controversy that has surrounded this disease through the whole history of medicine. The ancients were already faced with two concepts of the cause of *melancholy*. On the one hand, it was thought to be an organic disease due to invasion of the body in some mysterious way by a viscous, glutinous fluid, the *atra bilia*, the *black bile*. The cure, therefore, lay in giving medicine to drive out this fluid. On the other hand, there was the belief that a certain type of person with a "melancholic temperament" could become "melancholic" under certain circumstances as a result of external causes.

The doctors understandably inclined more to the first of these two concepts and treated their patients accordingly—though what success they had was probably mostly due to spontaneous healing. Today, psychopathology as well as clinical psychiatry still adheres to the concept of a single manic-depressive psychosis as postulated by Kraepelin. This is regarded as primarily constitutional and hereditary, and can thus be said to have a biological basis. Its various phases, which we perceive as illness, usually appear and disappear without obvious, or at least adequate, external cause. But the old philosophical ideas of melancholy still have their effect on our thinking. In the Middle Ages these concepts took literary, poetic and aesthetic forms. In this way, melancholy came to be associated with mourning for a personal loss or disappointment. Freud's treatise on *Mourning and Melancholy* and the psychoanalytical studies that followed it soon led to talk of a "psychogenesis" of melancholy. And so the old conflict was reintroduced into modern ideas and terminology, for now a distinction was made between "endogenous," "biological" and "reactive psychogenic" forms of depression, although admittedly the boundary between the two remained a fluctuating one.

A later further development was to play a significant role in the discovery of imipramine as antidepressive agent. In his outstanding contribution on "Endogenous and Reactive Depressions and the Manic-Depressive Constitution" in Bumke's treatise (Volume 6, Part 2, 1928), J. Lange drew a very important conclusion from Kraepelin's psychopathological ideas and his own clinical experience. On page 215, he writes:

> Opium appears to have a specific effect on melancholy, admittedly only a symptomatic one, and this is particularly striking because

opium itself causes some effects that resemble the symptoms of melancholy.

This statement led to a working hypothesis—namely, that it should be possible to find a drug acting in some specific manner against melancholy that is better than opium. It remained to be seen, of course, to what extent this substance would itself have effects resembling the disease.

It was now that the psychopathological recognition of this cyclic psychosis received a further and decisive impetus. This impetus came not, as one would in the nature of things have supposed, from biology or biochemistry, but, surprisingly enough, from philosophy. In the first decade of this century the work of K. Jaspers, combined with the philosophical trends of the time, prompted psychopathologists to look critically at their methods, at *what* they were actually doing in their field of psychopathology and *how* they were doing it. Like Jaspers, the Heidelberg school of the nineteen twenties, Kronfeld and Binswanger called on psychopathologists to make a fundamental distinction between the objective *behavior* and *performance* of the patient and his subjective *experiences* as they can be learned about from only his own description.

The so-called *phenomenological description* of pathological experiences made it possible for Kurt Schneider to apply to depression the doctrine of the philosopher Max Scheler in his work *The Stratification of the Emotional Life*, published in 1920. Schneider believed that this could help to explain and define the difference between endogenous and reactive depressions both clinically and phenomenologically by distinguishing the "*vital* feeling"—experienced as extending over the whole body by the patient with "endogenous, motiveless, psychotic depression" from the "*emotional* feeling"—likewise experienced but of a different nature—of the patient with "motivated depression of obvious cause."

It was on this basis that there arose the clearly defined syndrome of "vital depressive disturbance" with feelings of fatigue, lethargy, confinement, oppression and inhibition, accompanied by a slowing-down of thinking, acting and decision. This syndrome was marked by early-morning exacerbation and phases of alternating appearance and disappearance. Against this we have the "emotional depressive disturbance" marked by inability to feel pleasure and maintain interest or even by loss of the ability to experience any emotion whatsoever. Phenomenological analysis has greatly enriched the earlier psychopathological descriptions, in which disturbances of experience and behavior were not clearly distinguished. On the other hand, it soon became apparent, as Wyrsch, Binswanger and others pointed out, that vital disturbances are also a feature of motivated depressions, and thus of reactive depressions. Conversely, it was realized that endogenous depressions by no means leave the emotions untouched. With all this, however, the scientific psychopathological picture of the depressive states departs markedly from the naive concepts of melancholy as they were seen by traditional science. This has been made clear by long-term observations on patients with chronic reactive depressions, many of whom later exhibit endogenous phases. But before we pursue these interesting questions further, let me say a few words about *personal problems.*

A discovery does not arise of its own accord out of a particular scientific situation. There are many other factors at work. Among them there is one that probably plays a cardinal role—namely, the interaction of the researcher's scientific knowledge and practical observations with his personal experiences. However, this is a process that always defies full understanding and explanation.

As a schoolboy, I used to collect plants and believed that these or even just bright green water-colors could cure all sorts of dangerous diseases I had read or heard about. It is difficult to say what lay behind this childhood fantasy, but along with personal experience of illness and a general interest in human biology, it may well have played a role in my later decision to take up medicine. I must admit that my long-standing hope of discovering an effective drug received a severe set-back during my studies. Emil Bürgi, at that time an outstanding pharmacologist at the University of Berne, liked to warn his students about illusions of this sort: "Anybody who starts to look for a new hypnotic should be content if after years of work he ends up by finding a purgative." Bürgi had been trying for many years to prove his idea that the green pigment of plants had growth-promoting properties. What he failed to realize was that the effect of his preparations was diminished when they had been freed from carotene. His work came to an abrupt end with the discovery of vitamin A by other workers, an occasion that led him to make the bitter comment: "One can well ask oneself, why could all that not have succeeded with me?"

Bürgi's story of his bad luck always made a lasting impression on at least one of his students. It showed how immense are the difficulties surrounding the search for a new drug and at the same time how disastrous preconceived ideas can be.

As a young doctor, my choice of the psychiatric specialty, not entirely a deliberate one, offered only limited possibilities of using drug treatment. But what drugs there were I made very good use of. The main opportunity came with the treatment of psychosis by prolonged narcosis. This was in the Psychiatric Clinic in Berne, where Klaesi, the discoverer of the method, worked and taught. These so-called sleep cures were not without their dangers. They involved very close observation of the patient and of the effects of the narcotic used, so that patients often had to be visited day and night. This was before the time of the sulfonamides and antibiotics, and the risk of pneumonia was justly feared. It was essential to keep a constant watch on the patient's breathing, appearance and behavior so that the narcosis could be interrupted before the onset of physical signs and fever.

In addition to treating schizophrenia by prolonged narcosis, we used methiazole and electroshock, particularly for depressions. While the success of these methods can be said to have confirmed the biological basis of depression, they had a number of disagreeable features for not only the patient but also the doctor. On the one hand, they meant keeping the patients under close observation and always having to question them in order to avoid unnecessary treatment. On the other, they meant that efforts were made to find some drug whose simple administration could replace electroshock. The aim was a desirable one from another aspect. Intensive study of the literature on depressions and increasing experience were bringing to light more and more relatively mild cases of depressive disease. These were cases in which one was naturally disinclined to use the drastic method of electroshock, and the only other available method, the opium cure, while not entirely useless, was not effective enough.

HISTORY OF THE DISCOVERY

I come now to the story of the discovery itself. When the first psychopharmacological agents were discovered—chlorpromazine and the other phenothiazines that soon followed it—the question naturally arose of whether these substances might have an action on depressions superior to that of opium. After tests on a very few depressed patients, we found that the phenothiazines did indeed have a calming effect. But while this was occasionally accompanied by subjective alleviation of the patient's condition as well as an objective improvement in his behavior, these substances had no effect on the specific depressive symptoms.

What now happened may sound like an anecdote, but since it is part of the story, I must relate it. About 1950, Domenjoz of the firm of J. R. Geigy in Basel approached us with the request to try out one of their antihistamines [1] to see whether it could be used as a hypnotic. Although our tests turned out negative, it seemed to us that the substance had some special "antipsychotic" effects. However, the firm took no action on our suggestion to follow up these findings.

It was then that we heard of the effects of chlorpromazine, and before long we gathered some experience of our own. From this we got the impression that we had already seen the same or similar effects with Geigy's antihistamine. However, chlorpromazine turned out to be too expensive for the funds at our disposal in the quantities we needed, and this prompted us to remind Domenjoz about our earlier observations. On 17 February, 1954, we wrote a long letter to Geigy describing our experience with the antihistamine and the results we had obtained with chlorpromazine. Our letter again suggested that the antihistamine should be put to further clinical tests. This happened to be at the time when the firm had just resumed studies of this substance in relation to hibernation. The antihistamine had the code No. G 22150 and possessed the same ring system as imipramine together with a three-membered branched side chain. The substance had obvious psychopharmacological properties and, though these were difficult to determine precisely, they were clearly not the same as those of chlorpromazine. We soon found that it had no action on depressions. Moreover, its use on a large scale was impossible because of some disturbing side effects.

In conjunction with Domenjoz, we decided that the next substance of the group we would put to further clinical testing would be the one with the same side chain as chlorpromazine. This substance, No. G 22355, we tried out for about a year in various mental disorders and abnormalities. Little by little we gathered experience with it in about 300 cases. In order to reach a final verdict, we decided early in 1956 to test it on a number of patients with endogenous depressions, as we had already done with the previous preparation.

The really important decision we made here was not to pass a verdict on new psychopharmacological agents before we had tried them on patients with endogenous depressions. Thoroughness was not our only reason for doing this—there was also our conviction that it must be possible to find a drug effective in endogenous depressions. This conviction arose from the literature study I have already mentioned as well as from the great deal of experience we had acquired in the shock treatment of these depressions and in major psychotherapy of patients who presented with a neurosis but later turned out to be depressed.

After treating our first three cases, it was already clear to us that the substance G 22355, later known as imipramine, had an antidepressive action. On February 4, 1956, we sent Geigy a long report in which we pointed out the effect this substance had in depressions. Specifically, we said that if this finding were confirmed it would be of the utmost practical importance. Meanwhile, we pursued our clinical tests. At the Second International Congress of Psychiatry in Zurich on September 6, 1957, we reported the discovery in a paper read to an audience of barely a dozen people. The subject was dealt with in full in the issue of the *Swiss Medical Journal* of 31 August, 1957, devoted to the Congress.[2]

Our paper was received with some interest, but with a great deal of skepticism. This was not surprising in view of the almost completely negative history of the drug treatment of depression up to that time. Our conclusion that the substance had an antidepressive action was based on only 40 very closely studied cases. However, these were supported by our findings in 300 other patients.

FURTHER HISTORY OF THE DISCOVERY OF THE ANTIDEPRESSIVE EFFECT OF IMIPRAMINE

The true—I may say essential—significance of the discovery of imipramine came to be recognized only during the development of the drug treatment of depression in the years after 1957. I am not thinking here of the over 5,000 publications that have since appeared on imipramine and the substances derived from it, nor of the many millions of patients who have been treated with these drugs, nor of how it has helped them and the people around them, nor again of the purely material advantages of maintaining earning-power and avoiding hospitalization. No, I am thinking rather of the psychopathological, clinical, phramacological, biochemical and even purely chemical problems involved in the discovery of the imipramine effect. It is these that have done so much to further the recognition and understanding of depressive states and opened up the possibility of their treatment.

Let me first deal with the *clinical and pathological problems.* The first scientific description of the imipramine effect included all its main aspects, and even today there is nothing in it we would go back on. One statement in this report reads:

> The substance is particularly effective in typical endogenous depressions provided there is a vital disturbance standing clearly in the foreground.

As it later happened, we were mistaken in assuming that the expression "vital disturbance" was well understood. We expected that the average psychiatrist would be familiar with scientific ideas that had already been accepted for 25 years and would be guided by them in his diagnoses.

This experience revealed that there was world-wide ignorance of even Kraepelin's work at the beginning of this century, let alone that of Kurt Schneider and the later correction of his doctrine. It showed us the persistence of naive and popular concepts of the nature and outward appearance of "melancholy," that imipramine was being given to depressives who were tearful, distressed, despairing, self-accusing, plagued by feelings of guilt and sin and with suicidal tendencies. As was to be expected, the results obtained were not as good as in those cases where "*a vital disturbance was standing clearly in the foreground,*" where the patients complained of lassitude, feelings of heaviness, depression and inhibition, a slowing down and difficulty in thinking and acting, of internal tension and the inability to feel pleasure, the whole picture subject to diurnal fluctuations with exacerbation in the morning.

Further observation and experiment—to some extent prompted by outside criticism—convinced us more and more that the indication for antidepressives of the imipramine type lies in the phenomenological study of the subjective *experiences* of the patient, in the vital and emotional depressive disturbance. The *behavior* of the depressed patient is very strongly affected by external factors, by peculiarities of character and by the often widely fluctuating admixture of manic symptoms. Thus in addition to the inhibited, anxious and excited depressive, we have not only the tearful depressive but the smiling depressive with his "gallows humor." But above all, as Freud long ago stated, depressive features are to be found in nearly all neuroses. The more a psychopathological condition or attitude is affected from its inception by depressive experiences, or the more evident such experiences become, the better are the chances of successful treatment with an antidepressive drug, whether in support of psychotherapy or as a substitute for it. Indeed, apart from continued psychotherapeutic counseling, further psychotherapy may in many cases be rendered superfluous.

The questions of outward *behavior* in depression and of the endogenous or reactive psychogenic *origin* of depression—both still regarded today as the decisive diagnostic criteria—have thus largely been pushed into the background. At the same time, another factor has emerged, namely the *stress of daily life* at home and at work, together with what we might call "buffetings of fate." The less exacting a person's daily life is, the less a depression manifests itself, and vice versa. This is the reason why hospitalization often brings about a marked improvement in depressive symptoms. In our opinion, therefore, it is wise never to give a final verdict on a new antidepressive agent that has been tested on only patients in hospital. Only the patient who has to cope with the vicissitudes of daily life can show clearly whether and to what extent any new substance really has an antidepressive action.

The difficulty is that it is not very easy to select from the many available patients suitable ones for antidepressive treatment. On the one hand, it is difficult to judge how heavy the burdens of daily life are; on the other, in only a few patients is the diagnosis obvious or easily made from statements by the patient's family. Many patients recount absolutely nothing spontaneously about their depressive experiences, and these come to light only on questioning. Even then, the patient may deny the experiences and admit to them, and describe them, only retrospectively when his condition has improved.

It has at last been recognized that the vital depressive disturbance can often be traced back to childhood. Children are even less inclined to relate their emotional experiences spontaneously or describe them when asked. The psychiatrist must depend here on the heredity and on what he can learn from the parents concerning any obvious change of mood or particular type of behavior. We know that the latter differs widely from the average psychiatrist's idea of how depressives behave. It is above all the morning mood that provides important indicators. We know too about the child whose sluggish and tearful behavior is often mistaken for laziness, the picture of the infantile stage of melancholy so impressively described by Shakespeare in *As You Like It.* The symptoms are sleeplessness, anxiety, tiredness and thus failure at school in spite of high intelligence, neglect of school homework, the "sitting in front of a blank page" because the child can think of nothing to write. Other common symptoms are playing hooky, enuresis and encopresis; in short, many that are today still interpreted by child psychiatrists as due to environmental damage, poor upbringing, or neurosis.

I now come to the *pharmacological, biochemical and chemical aspects.* The introduction of imipramine as an antidepressive agent by the firm of Geigy in the spring of 1958 brought a disappointment in that the side effects were manifestly more troublesome than our original studies had suggested. At first this remained a mystery, but in the course of the next few years it was largely explained. Most of the side effects are neurovegetative disturbances due to upsets and functional overloading of the autonomic nervous system. They, therefore, depend on the intervals between doses of the drug, on the time of the day it is taken, on the relation to meals, and on physical and mental strain. For this reason, the side effects are much less serious in hospitalized patients than in those who have to cope with the stresses of daily life.

The problem of side effects comprises an important part of the pharmacology of imipramine and indeed of antidepressives in general.[3] As far as we know, depression does not occur in animals, or is at least not demonstrable, so that the pharmacological pattern seen in animal studies is much more that of the side effects than the pattern seen when depressed patients are treated. Unlike other investigators, we have always been of the opinion that at least the neurovegetative and extrapyramidal effects are true side effects and distinguishable clearly from the specific antidepressive components. For this reason, we suggested that Geigy should let us test some substances with a less marked pharmacological profile. Among them was a preparation that in animal experiments had shown fewer qualities regarded as typical of antidepressive agents and, in particular, had no atropine activity. The result was the discovery of the excellent antidepressive properties of ketimipramine, in which the carbon bridge has a keto group and which is largely free of side effects even in ambulant patients.

Here I cannot go into the many interesting consequences of these studies. Nor have I time to deal with the hypothetical and actual relationships between antidepressive and sedative activity, which among other things led to the development of amitriptyline and its derivatives. Suffice it for me to say that we hold the view that an ideal antidepressive agent should possess no sedative activity. Metabolic studies of imipramine have given results of great practical utility. On the other hand, no useful conclusions have yet been drawn from the effect of the drug on adrenergic synapses.

Both biological considerations in general and clinical experience suggest looking for connections between chemical structure and activity. So far it seems that various factors determine antidepressive action. An important part appears to be played by the angle between the rings in the system.[4] Thus the first clinical tests of an octadiene derivative of Ciba in Basel showed the antidepressive activity we had anticipated from the presence of this angle and other stereochemical characteristics, and indeed to a very remarkable extent.[5]

This is as far as I can go in telling you the Imipramine Story, not because it has come to an end but because it brings us up to the present, so to speak into the laboratory of the clinical pharmacologist as well as that of the discoverer himself. Ketimipramine will not completely replace imipramine, but it will probably bring about a big improvement in antidepressive treatment, particularly of ambulant patients. The octadiene derivative I mentioned is a completely new antidepressive agent with an activity spectrum extending in the direction of schizophrenia. (It is the substance that our friend Bein discussed here yesterday from the pharmacologic point of view; he has told you this part of the tricyclic antidepressant story.) Both substances have a future, but what this will bring is still speculation. However, we foresee possible further developments with very important consequences.

This prospect brings me to a final consideration. What lessons does the Imipramine Story have for us? What Lange has already said about opium probably applies to a much greater extent to imipramine and some of its derivatives. We have achieved a *specific* treatment of depressive states, not ideal but already going far in this direction. I emphasize "specific" because the drug largely or completely restores what the illness has impaired—namely, the mental functions and capacity and what is of prime importance, the power to experience. Specific, too, because withdrawal of the treatment when the disease is active results in reappearance of the symptoms just as they were before treatment was started.

However, this is true only if one condition is fulfilled—namely, that we are prepared to recognize a particular pathological picture in which the drug is in fact successful. Now this is a picture only partly coinciding with the classic clinical idea of the depressive states. In fact, it goes a good deal further than this, for it embraces chronic as well as phasic disturbances, certain organic, schizoid-schizophrenic and reactive as well as endogenous disturbances. Moreover, it is to a considerable extent subject to the phenomenological description of vital and emotional experiences. What I am endeavoring to say is that the essence of the discovery of imipramine has been the elaboration of a particular clinical disease picture that allows us to choose exactly those patients who will benefit from the drug from among the great mass of persons who are mentally ill. It is in this connection that some doctors, who tested imipramine with no particular idea of its possible activity, failed, and they considered it useless. But many doctors today are still incapable of making use of imipramine simply because they have preconceived notions of what a depression looks like and how it should be assessed, and because they largely or entirely neglect the patient's own experiences. *If* we are to use the important drugs in the antidepressive group successfully, we must also learn to recognize something new, indeed to *discover* something never before seen or recognized.

Chance admittedly had something to do with the discovery of imipramine. Chance was not decisive, however, even though the discoverer was privileged to turn this chance to good account. Good fortune, too, played a part, but to this had to be added a measure of *intellectual achievement* that was able to "invent" something completely new, something hitherto unknown, namely a new disease. As I hope I have been able to make more or less clear to you today, the discovery of the antidepressive properties of imipramine thus appears not only as a unique event, as a lucky chance, but also an achievement of the progressively developing human intellect, with its manifold limitations and freedoms. Goethe put the essence of the matter in a nutshell when he wrote: "Discovery needs luck, invention, intellect—neither can do without the other."

REFERENCES

1. Schindler, W., and Häfliger, F.: Helv Chim Acta *37*:427, 1954.
2. Kuhn, R.: Schweiz med Wschr *87*:1135, 1957.
3. Domenjoz, R., and Theobald, W.: Arch Int Pharmacodyn *120*:450, 1959.
4. Häfliger, F.: Canad Psychiat Ass *4*:S 69, 1959.
5. Kuhn, R.: Proceedings of the VI Intn Congr of the CINP—Excerpta Med Intern Congr Series No. 180, 1968, pp. 512-513.

CHAPTER

17

The Story of Lithium

John F. J. Cade, MD, FANZCP *

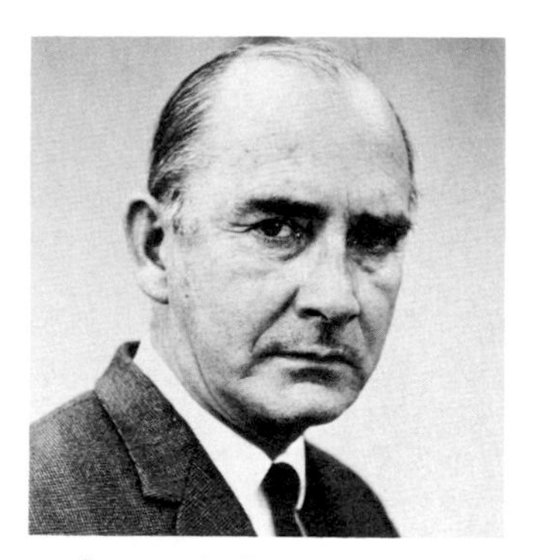

Lithium has had an erratic history in medicine. The alkali metal itself was discovered by Arfvedson in 1817, whilst analyzing the mineral petalite. Chemically it resembles sodium and potassium. It decomposes water, but the hydrogen does not ignite as it does with the other two. It is widely distributed in small quantities and has been detected in sea water and many spring and river waters, in the ash of many plants, in various animal organs and even in meteorites.

Lithium salts were introduced into medicine by A. B. Garrod in 1859 for the treatment of gout, following the demonstration that lithium urate was the most soluble of the urates.[4] It was shown that if pieces of cartilage with urate deposits were immersed in solutions of sodium, potassium and lithium carbonate, the urate was dissolved first from that piece immersed in the lithium carbonate solution.

As time went on and lithia tablets were consumed on an ever-increasing scale for an ever-increasing range of ailments, the toxic effects were more and more commonly seen. In *The Practitioner* in 1907 cases were reported "of cardiac depression and even dilation, as a result of excessive and continued consumption of lithia tablets." [5] It was also recorded that "lithia salts upset the stomach very easily." [6]

Culbreth (1927) stated that lithium bromide is the most hypnotic

* President, Australian and New Zealand College of Psychiatrists; Senior Associate in Psychiatry, Examiner in Psychological Medicine, University of Melbourne.

of all bromides (and almost certainly it would be).[3] The recommended dose was the relatively enormous one of 10 to 30 grains (600 to 1,800 mg). It is not stated how often this dose might be repeated each day, but no doubt most would assume that it could be prescribed the traditional twice or thrice daily. As 15 grains (900 mg) of lithium bromide repeated three times a day would soon lead not only to bromide but to the far more dangerous lithium intoxication, it is little wonder that it never found favor in the treatment of epilepsy.

It is worth noting that the hypnotic action of lithium bromide was thought to be due to the fact that, the atomic weight of lithium being so small, weight for weight, lithium bromide must contain more bromide than any other bromide salt. There is no evidence that the lithium ion was recognized as having any psychotropic action itself. What with the toxic effects of laissez-faire administration and the uselessness of lithium in most of the conditions for which it was prescribed, it is not surprising that lithium salts fell into disuse.

But worse was to come. They fell into active and unfortunately justified disrepute. In the 1940's, lithium chloride was used as a sodium chloride substitute in an uncontrolled way in attempts to combat the edema of congestive cardiac failure—with the inevitable disastrous consequences. Deaths were being reported in the *Journal of the American Medical Association* in 1949. The *JAMA* of 12 March that year (1949) sounded the death knell of the reputation of lithium with two papers, a case report and a letter emphasizing its toxicity. But of course it was used in quite the wrong way for the treatment of precisely those patients in whom its use is positively contraindicated.

One can hardly imagine a less propitious year in which to attempt the pharmacological rehabilitation of lithium. That the attempt was made by an unknown psychiatrist, working alone in a small chronic hospital with no research training, primitive techniques and negligible equipment was hardly likely to be compellingly persuasive, especially in the United States. And so it turned out. It is a source of singular satisfaction to me that after the lapse of years the therapeutic and theoretical importance of lithium has at last been recognized. The person who has done most to achieve this recognition by validating and extending my original observations has been Mogens Schou in Denmark.

My discovery of the specific antimanic effect of the lithium ion was an unexpected but, to be retrospectively percipient for a moment, inevitable by-product of experimental work I was doing to test a hypothesis regarding the etiology of manic-depressive illness. Could it be analogous to thyrotoxicosis and myxedema, mania being a state of intoxication by a normal product of the body circulating in excess, whilst melancholia is the corresponding deprivative condition? If this hypothesis is accepted as a working basis for investigation, it is evident that the key to the problem lies in the study of the manic patient who is assumed to be producing the intoxicating substance in excess and may well be excreting it in the urine. The first step then was to attempt to devise a method of demonstrating such a toxic agent, if it existed, in the urine of manic patients. Because I did not know what the substance might be, still less anything of its pharmacology for lower animals, the best plan seemed to be to spread the net as wide as possible and use the crudest form of biological test in a preliminary investigation.

For this purpose, guinea pigs were used and fresh urine was injected intraperitoneally. Using concentrated urine (the early morning specimen passed after abstinence from fluid for 12 to 14 hours), it soon became evident that some specimens of urine from manic patients were far more toxic than any of the control specimens from normal persons, schizophrenics and melancholics. The urine from some manic patients would kill the animals in as low a dose as 0.25 ml per 30 Gm body weight, whereas the most toxic control specimen was not lethal in doses lower than 0.75 ml per 30 Gm body weight. All that had been demonstrated so far was that any concentrated urine in sufficient quantity would kill a guinea pig, but that urine from a manic subject often killed much more readily.

Now the mode of death is the same in all cases, manic and control, suggesting that the same toxic agent is at work. After a latent period of 12 to 28 minutes, in which the animal appears perfectly well, apart from occasional initial distress of a few minutes following the injection, it becomes tremulous and ataxic, and in a few minutes quadriplegic, the hind legs being the first affected. It remains fully conscious and often squeals when picked up at this stage. Myoclonic twitching precedes a severe tonic convulsion, and from then on the animal remains unconscious in status epilepticus of tonic type with convulsive gasping until its death a few or many minutes later. An occasional animal recovers.

In an attempt to identify the actual toxic agent in the urine the principal end products of nitrogenous metabolism were first investigated. It was not very surprising to find that urea was the guilty substance. In a 4% aqueous solution its lethal dose for guinea pigs was 1.0 to 1.25 mg per 30 Gms of body weight, a relatively enormous dose, roughly equivalent to 100 Gms in a 70 Kg man. The mode of death was exactly the same as with urine. An interesting point is that there appear to be no intermediate effects. The animal either develops no symptoms whatever following the injection or it dies. Uric acid 0.1% solution in normal saline and creatinine 0.1% solution in normal saline appeared to have no toxic effects at all when injected intraperitoneally in maximal doses. It is impossible to inject more than about 2 ml of fluid per 30 Gm of body weight into the peritoneal cavity of a guinea pig.

Although the actual toxic agent was identified, this was only a first step. The next was to identify the quantitative modifiers that made some specimens of urine from manics so much more toxic than any specimen from other sources. It was not simply that these more toxic urines contained a higher concentration of urea. As the lethal dose of a 4% aqueous solution of urea is about 1 ml per 30 Gm body weight, one would have to postulate an impossible concentration of 8 to 16% urea in these specimens. In fact quantitative estimations showed that urine from manic subjects did not differ significantly from that of nonmanics or controls in urea content.

Were uric acid or creatinine the quantitative modifiers? Uric acid has a slight effect in enhancing the toxicity of urea, but the most surprising observation was the remarkable protective action of creatinine. The minimal lethal dose of an aqueous solution of 0.025% creatinine and 4% urea is double that of a 4% solution urea only. The same degree of protection is afforded by a fairly wide range of creatinine concentrations; 0.025% gives as much protection as 0.2% and more than counterbalances the mildly enhancing toxic effect of uric acid.

Creatinine is also strongly protective against the convulsive and lethal effects of cardiazol (Pentamethylenetetrazol). In 10% solution, an intraperitoneal injection of 0.015 ml per 30 Gms body weight produces in guinea pigs merely mild transient myoclonic twitching, commencing one to two minutes after injection and lasting several minutes. Twice this dose is fatal. In one to two minutes, there is severe myoclonus quickly developing into a furious clonic fit. The animals go into a status epilepticus of clonic type and die three-quarters to one hour later. An intraperitoneal injection of 9.5% aqueous solution of creatinine in a dose of 0.33 ml per 30 Gm given 25 minutes before an otherwise lethal dose of 0.03 ml of Cardiazol per 30 Gm body weight results in a 50% reduction in mortality and a 25% suppression of convulsive phenomena. Creatinine itself appears to have no toxic effects even in comparatively huge doses.

In brief, the situation at this stage was as follows: the toxicity of some specimens of urine from manic patients was considerably more than could be explained on the assumption that the protective action of creatinine had been simply neutralized. The specimens were more toxic than could be explained by the concentrations of urea actually present even if the urea effect were being maximally enhanced by uric acid. It is difficult to avoid postulating a third substance in such specimens that more than neutralizes the powerful protective action of creatinine. Further it is disappointing to record that this hypothetical enhancer of urea toxicity has not been identified.

It now appeared important to estimate more accurately how much uric acid increased the toxicity of urea. The practical difficulty was the comparative insolubility of uric acid in water, so the most soluble urate was chosen—the lithium salt. And that is how lithium came into the story.

When an aqueous solution of 8% urea, saturated with lithium urate was injected, the toxicity was far less than expected. It appeared as if the lithium ion may have been exerting a protective effect. More observations were made, lithium carbonate being used instead of lithium urate. An 8% aqueous solution of urea kills five out of 10 guinea pigs when injected intraperitoneally in doses of 1.25 ml per 30 Gm body weight. When 0.5% lithium carbonate in an 8% urea solution was injected in the same dose, all the animals survived. This argues for a strong protective function for the lithium ion against the convulsant mode of death produced by toxic doses of urea.

To determine whether lithium salts by themselves had any discernible effects on guinea pigs, animals were injected intraperitoneally with large doses of 0.5% aqueous solution of lithium carbonate. A noteworthy result was that after a latent period of about two hours the animals, although fully conscious, became extremely lethargic and unresponsive to stimuli for one to two hours before once again becoming normally timid and active. Those who have experimented with guinea pigs know to what degree a ready startle reaction is part of their make-up. It was thus even more startling to the experimenter to find that after the injection of a solution of lithium carbonate they could be turned on their backs and that, instead of their usual frantic righting reflex behavior, they merely lay there and gazed placidly back at him.

It may seem a long way from lethargy in guinea pigs to the control of manic excitement, but as these investigations had commenced in an attempt to demonstrate some possibly excreted toxin in the urine of manic patients, the association of ideas is explicable. As lithium salts had been in use in medical practice since the middle of the nineteenth century, albeit in a haphazard way with negligible therapeutic results, there seemed no ethical contraindications to using them in mania, especially as single and repeated doses of lithium citrate and lithium carbonate in the doses contemplated produced no discernible ill effects on the investigator himself.

Originally, two alternative salts were used—the citrate because of its solubility but increasingly the carbonate because it is better tolerated and much less likely to produce alimentary disturbances. The original therapeutic dose decided on fortuitously proved to be the optimum, that is 1,200 mg of the citrate thrice daily or 600 mg of the carbonate. For years now we have used the carbonate exclusively in 300 mg tablets. Once normal emotional tone is attained, the dose is progressively reduced to maintenance medication of 300 to 900 mg daily, six days a week.

In my first paper (Cade, 1949), I described the results of treatment of 10 manic patients, six schizophrenics and three chronic psychotic depressives.[1]

As this is an historical symposium, you may be interested in the case report of the very first manic patient ever deliberately and successfully treated with lithium salts. This was a little wizened man of 51 who had been in a state of chronic manic excitement for five years. He was amiably restless, dirty, destructive, mischievous and interfering. He had enjoyed preeminent nuisance value in a back ward for all those years and bid fair to remain there for the rest of his life.

He commenced treatment with lithium citrate 1200 mg tid on 29 March, 1948. On the fourth day, the optimistic therapist thought he saw some change for the better but acknowledged that it could have been his expectant imagination; the nursing staff were non-committal but loyal. However, by the fifth day it was clear that he was in fact more settled, tidier, less disinhibited and less distractible. From then on there was steady improvement so that in three weeks he was enjoying the unaccustomed and quite unexpected amenities of a convalescent ward. As he had been ill so long and confined to a chronic ward he found normal surroundings and liberty of movement strange at first. Owing to this, as well as housing difficulties and the necessity of determining a satisfactory maintenance dose, he was kept under observation for two months. He remained perfectly well and left hospital on 9 July, 1948, on indefinite leave with instructions to take a maintenance dose of lithium carbonate, 300 mg bid. The carbonate had been substituted for the citrate as he had become intolerant of the latter, complaining of severe nausea. He was soon back working happily at his old job. However, he became more lackadaisical about his medicine and finally ceased taking it. His relatives reported that he had not had any for at least six weeks prior to his readmission six months later and was becoming steadily more irritable and erratic. His lithium carbonate was at once recommenced, 600 mg thrice daily and in two weeks he had again returned to normal. The dose was then reduced to 300 mg thrice daily and in another two weeks to 300 mg twice daily. A month later he is recorded as completely well and ready to return to home and work.

The results with the other nine manic patients were equally gratifying. In the light of subsequent developments and observations, the report of the tenth patient's response is interesting. These days he would be described as schizoaffective. He was in an excited, euphoric hallucinatory delusional state. It was noted at the time that the excitement was well controlled by lithium but that the delusional state was quite unaffected.

Of the six schizophrenic patients treated, an important observation was that although there was no fundamental improvement in any of them, three who were usually restless, noisy and shouting nonsensical abuse, like the schizoaffective patient, lost their excitement and restlessness and became quiet and amenable for the first time in years. Taking a nocturnal hypnotic had been a routine and could be discontinued during treatment. They reverted to their previous state on cessation of lithium medication.

In three chronically depressed patients, lithium produced neither amelioration nor aggravation of their symptoms. That, then, is the story of the launching of lithium as a specific antimanic drug.

Following this initial discovery my interests have taken two different paths:

> *1/* The further evaluation of lithium and the identification of significant cation distributions in functional psychoses. This has culminated in some fascinating recent work in my own hospital that will be the subject of another paper. Suffice it to say that we are now able to identify, on the basis of a simple lithium excretion test, those who are likely to be lithium responders, irrespective of symptomatic presentation. This work bids fair to cut across the whole of contemporary nosology.
>
> *2/* Second, it was inevitable, having thus been unexpectedly presented with a therapeutic magic wand, that one would plunge one's hand time and again into the same lucky dip. It is this work I now propose to discuss and briefly to review other nontoxic cations that over the years I have screened for possible psychotropic activity. It must be emphasized that this work has been desultory and involved the crudest experimental techniques so that any positive observations must be subject to confirmation and any conclusions tentative.

As lithium has such a pronounced psychotropic effect, it might be expected that salts of *rubidium* and *caesium* (the other alkali metals in addition to sodium and potassium) might also. Single doses in guinea pigs and later repeated doses in rats had no discernible effects even in comparatively huge doses, i.e. the equivalent of 100 Gm of rubidium chloride in a 70 Kg man over a period of five days.

Cerium salts injected intraperitoneally in rats produce a marked anergic state developing within three to five minutes and lasting about two hours. The animals remain awake but motionless, responding only reluctantly to stimulation, such as pinching the tip of the tail. The righting reflex remains but is feeble, and they are so anergic that they are unable to hop back into their cages. Respiration is markedly slowed–i.e., to about 100 per minute or about half the normal rate. The animal feels atonic when held in the hand and protests little when held belly upward.

An attempt was made to identify the active agent responsible for this "cerium effect," as cerium salts are generally very impure, containing appreciable quantities (up to 10%) of the other rare earths, lanthanum, neodymium and praesodymium, and one of these rather than the cerium might have been responsible. They are chemically so similar that they are extremely difficult to separate. It might be predicted that they would all show the same sort of pharmacological behavior. I was fortunate in being able to obtain from the Department of Chemistry of the University of Melbourne some relatively pure samples. Briefly the results were as follows:

Lanthanum produced a similar but if anything slightly stronger response than cerium. *Neodymium* behaved exactly the same as cerium, but—surprisingly in view of the chemical similarity of all four—*praesodymium* produced no discernible effect of this kind. As far as the responsible agent is concerned, it does not really matter whether an impure salt of cerium is used because the impurities produce either the same effect (lanthanum and neodymium) or no effect at all (praesodymium). Cerium carbonate given orally to rats 600 mg daily incorporated in food pellets for 14 days in young female rats produced no discernible effect.

As cerium is not a biological poison (the oxalate was prescribed up till the 1894 edition of the British Pharmacopoeia as a remedy for sea sickness and hyperemesis gravidarum and has been described in the American, Japanese and Mexican Pharmacopoeias), I ascertained that cerium carbonate in 1,200 mg doses produces no dyspepsia and up to 4,800 mg daily had no discernible effect on me. But neither did it have the slightest therapeutic effect in doses of 900 mg thrice daily for at least a week in four psychotic patients—two psychotic depressives, one manic and one chronic paranoid schizophrenic. There the matter rests. Cerium salts, although having a marked sedative effect on intraperitoneal injection in rats, seem to have no psychopharmacological effect when orally administered in man.

The "cerium effect" is of course quite different from the sedative effect of lithium. With the former, the effect is evident in a few minutes and is wearing off after two hours, whereas lithium's effect is only starting to become evident after about two hours.

Strontium. The only other cation that I have looked at that seems to have any sort of psychotropic interest and possible therapeutic value, apart from lithium, is strontium. It might be asked why I chose to evaluate it at all. It was not simply that I was working my way systematically through the periodic table. I had already shown (Cade 1964) that plasma magnesium levels are considerably higher (35-40%) in severely depressed patients than in normal controls.[2] This result was significant at better than 1% level of probability. It seemed reasonable therefore to determine how psychotic depressives handle the magnesium ion. In brief, melancholics retain rather than excrete a loading dose of a magnesium salt as compared with controls, who react with a prompt increase in both Mg and Ca excretion. With schizophrenics the results were intermediate between the significant differences between melancholics and controls, but were not at the level of statistical significance.

Considering possible therapeutic intervention in the light of these findings, if the simple hypothesis that melancholia is related to magnesium retention has any validity, then the obvious lines of thought are reduction of magnesium ingestion and absorption, and promotion of magnesium excretion. Another less obvious approach, analogous to the use of lithium salts in mania, would be to discover whether another divalent cation by perhaps interfering with or substituting for the magnesium ion had any psychotropic effect.

Strontium salts were chosen for trial *1/* because it is becoming increasingly clear from recent work that Sr^{++} competes with Mg^{++} and Ca^{++} for paths of intestinal absorption and renal tubular excretion, *2/* because Sr^{++} may interfere with or modify Ca^{++} or Mg^{++} mediated metabolism, and *3/* because various strontium salts have been quite widely used in medicine (although they have long since disappeared from the British Pharmacopoeia) and there appears to be no record of toxic effects attributable to them. As with lithium, no one was interested in the cation. It was merely another vehicle to carry what was esteemed to be the appropriate active anion for the particular illness.

Strontium carbonate was chosen for use because it is the least likely to produce alimentary disturbance and because the anion is devoid of psychotropic effects. The first step was to decide an appropriate dose schedule from the points of view of both tolerance and side effects. Up to 4 Gms in a single dose produced no undesirable, indeed discernible, alimentary or systemic effects. Ingested 4 Gms thrice daily after meals for five days, i.e., a total of 60 Gms, there was no alimentary disturbance. The general effects noted were:

1/ a distinct tranquilizing effect. I am not a tension-prone individual, but I was under considerable irritating stress that week and was surprised by my equanimity under the circumstances.

2/ some heaviness and slight headache at times.

3/ by the fifth day, considerable drowsiness but not sufficient to interfere with work efficiency. However, on the next day, a holiday and the first day after discontinuance, I spent most of the day dozing. Thereafter, nothing further was noted.

As it had a tranquilizing and mildly sedative effect on such a relatively pharmacologically tough animal as myself, it seemed reasonable to evaluate it further, and over 10 months its effect on over 30 patients suffering from a variety of psychiatric disorders was assessed. There is no doubt whatever that it is substantially anxiolytic, safe, effective, and cheap. Even in patients who showed no real improvement otherwise, there was in many cases a tranquilizing effect with diminished restlessness and in some, drowsiness. In the two patients with anxiety severe enough to warrant hospitalization, there was complete and prompt remission in two days. In seven acute schizophrenics, there was complete and prompt remission in four, substantial symptomatic improvement in another, and in two no effect whatever.

Unfortunately, we do not know the spontaneous remission rate of acute schizophrenic reactions because such patients are almost invariably subjected to physical treatment of one kind or another almost from the moment they arrive in the ward. It was interesting, however, to observe the time interval between commencement of treatment and remission in both the schizophrenics and the two manics who remitted: they all remitted between the sixth and the eighth day. Most would agree that this is tenuous evidence on which to base any sort of therapeutic claim and I wholeheartedly concur. I merely present the results as interesting, possibly significant, certainly worthy of further study.

In the third manic patient, the result was nil apart from the tranquilizing effect, which she bitterly resented because the salt acted as a pharmacological restraint on her exuberance. When discontinued, it had to be replaced with thioridazine 200 mg thrice daily to keep her within practical nursing bounds, and this may be accepted as the approximate phenothiazine equivalent of 4 Gms of strontium carbonate thrice daily. This patient, by the way, responded perfectly satisfactorily to lithium.

In two severe psychotic depressives, the result was nil. It was considered unjustifiable to proceed further with such patients in view of the fact that adequate antidepressant treatment exists. In ten chronic schizophrenics the results were nil apart from a mild to moderate nonspecific tranquilizing effect in four.

Side effects. Anorexia, nausea, and vomiting are relatively common with medication at the maximum level of 4 Gms tid pc. It subsides quickly with temporary reduction or cessation of dosage. One of the 31 patients developed a Stevens-Johnson syndrome. It is quite impossible to say whether it was merely coincidental, but it must certainly be recorded. It remitted with adequate steroid dosage and antibiotic cover. Intraperitoneal injection of solutions of strontium chloride into rats and guinea pigs in doses comparable with those used orally in human beings produces mild sedation and considerable diminution of their startle response, confirming the validity of the tranquilizing effect observed in man.

To conclude I should like to emphasize these points:

> That lithium, a simple inorganic ion, can reverse a major psychotic reaction must have, quite apart from its substantial therapeutic value, profound theoretical significance in unraveling the mystery of the so-called functional psychoses. It must be regarded as a major research tool. Strontium may also prove to have a similar value for research in this field even if it has only minor therapeutic value.

REFERENCES

1. Cade, J. F. J.: Lithium salts in the treatment of psychotic excitement, Med J Aust *1*:195, 1949.

2. ——: A significant elevation of plasma magnesium levels in schizophrenia and depressive states, Med J Aust *1*:195, 1964.

3. Culbreth, D. M. R.: Materia Medica and Pharmacology, ed. 7, 1927, p. 743.

4. Garrod, A. B.: Gout and Rheumatic Gout, London, Walton and Maberly, 1859, p. 438.

5. The Practitioner: Quoted in Squire's Companion to British Pharmacopoeia, vol. 1, 1907, p. 116.

6. ——: Quoted by Squire, loco citato, vol. 2, 1909, p. 130.

CHAPTER

18

The Impact of Biological Psychiatry

FRANK J. AYD, JR., MD, FAPA*

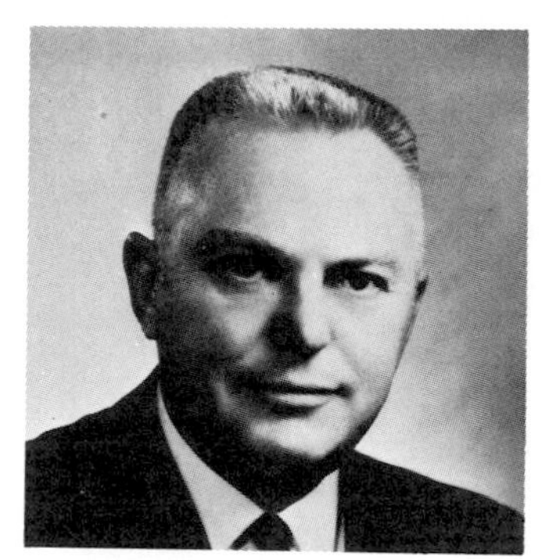

THE HISTORY OF TWENTIETH-CENTURY psychiatry makes an exciting narrative of the evolution of psychodynamic and physical methods of treatment; of therapeutic nihilism yielding to a spirit of expectant optimism; of a struggle against prejudice, inertia, and indifference; of the blossoming of multidisciplinary scientific interest in mental illness; of an unprecedented availability of money and manpower for psychiatric research; and of remarkable strides forward in the conquest of diseases of the mind.

The chemical revolution in psychiatry began in the early 1950s with the initial announcements on chlorpromazine and reserpine treatment of emotional and mental aberrations. These drugs were heralded as safe therapeutic agents, which radically altered the treatment, the course, and the prognosis of various psychiatric ailments. Psychiatric hospitals reported a decrease in the use of physical restraints, seclusion rooms, hydrotherapy, shock therapies, and other somatic methods of treatment; a reduction in destructiveness, combativeness, and assaultiveness; a greater number of ground privileges; and, above all, an increase in the discharge rate, especially of chronic patients who previously had been considered hopeless cases, and by some as "the living dead." Private practicing psychiatrists claimed that, properly used, these drugs increased the number of patients who could be treated in the office, facilitated psychotherapy, and made hospitalization unnecessary in many

* Editor: *The International Drug Therapy Newsletter.*

cases, thereby decreasing the number of admissions to overcrowded public mental hospitals and reducing the cost of psychiatric care.

The therapeutic successes with chlorpromazine and reserpine stimulated an intensive search for additional psychopharmaceuticals. This produced not only more neuroleptics, phenothiazines, thioxanthenes, and butyrophenones, but minor tranquilizers, of which meprobamate was the first, and equally important for the millions who suffer from melancholia, antidepressants, such as imipramine and amitriptyline. And because medical progress will not be checked, additional tranquilizers and antidepressants have been and will be developed by the pharmaceutical industry. The tranquilizers and antidepressants now available have made it possible for all physicians, not just psychiatrists, to treat their emotionally and mentally disturbed patients—something previously not possible.

In the past seventeen years, psychotropic drugs have been used for the treatment of at least 500,000,000 patients around the world. A concise review of what has been accomplished and what we have learned from this extensive clinical experience is the objective of this chapter.

WHAT HAS BEEN ACCOMPLISHED

To appreciate the unprecedented advances since the advent of chemopsychiatry, it is necessary to recall what conditions were like in the predrug era. There were few outpatient clinics and no day and night hospitals and community mental health centers as there are now. Despite the prevalence of psychiatrically ill patients, more than half of the general hospitals in the United States would not admit a known psychiatric patient, one-third admitted such patients solely for diagnosis or emergency treatment, and only one per cent had a psychiatric service primarily for short-term treatment. An attitude of pessimism and despair toward mental illness was prevalent.

Because of a lack of effective therapies, each year the national increment to the mental hospital population rose steadily. Within the bare walls of isolated, overcrowded, prison-like asylums were housed many screaming, combative individuals whose animalistic behavior required restraint and seclusion. Catatonic patients stood day after day, rigid as statues, their legs swollen and bursting with dependent edema. Their comrades idled week after week, lying on hard benches or the floor, deteriorating, aware only of their delusions and hallucinations. Others were incessantly restive, pacing back and forth like caged animals in a zoo. Periodically the air was pierced by the shouts of a raving patient. Suddenly, without notice, like an erupting volcano, an anergic schizophrenic bursts into frenetic behavior, lashing out at others or striking himself with his fists, or running wildly and aimlessly about.

Nurses and attendants, ever in danger, spent their time protecting patients from harming themselves or others. They watched men and women who either refused to eat or gorged themselves. They tube-fed to sustain life. Trained to be therapists, they functioned as guards and custodians in a hellish environment where despair prevailed and surcease by death offered the only lasting respite for their suffering charges.

Compounding this ghastly situation was the restricted therapeutic armamentarium of the psychiatrists. How frustrated and impotent they felt as they watched the number of chronically ill swell the burgeoning population of long-term resident patients. They knew from bitter experience that psychotherapy for psychotics was fruitless, that insulin coma and electroshock therapy offered little or no improvement to schizophrenics continuously ill for more than two years, and that psychosurgery benefited only a very small percentage of the chronically ill. For lack of more effective remedies, they secluded dangerously frenetic individuals behind thick doors in barred rooms stripped of all furniture and lacking toilet facilities. They restrained many others in cuffs and jackets or chained them to floors and walls. Daily they sent patients for hydrotherapy, where they were immersed for long hours in tubs, or were packed in wet sheets until their disturbed behavior subsided. These measures, barbaric and inhumane as they appear in retrospect, euphemistically called therapy, at best offered protection to patient and personnel and a temporary respite from the most distressing symptoms of psychoses.

This lack of effective antipsychotic therapies accounted for the bleak outlook for the chronically ill. Unless they were released within two to three years of admission, they were destined to remain indefinitely, prisoners of psychoses—unresponsive to the existing therapies.

By 1955, because of the therapeutic effectiveness of the psychotropic drugs, psychiatric hospitals became able to discharge patients at an unprecedented rate. In 1956, for the first time in 175 years, the number of patients in the United States psychiatric hospitals began to decline. Each year since, despite a steady increase in the admission rate, there has been a substantial decrease in the resident population of mental hospitals to an all time low of approximately 400,000 patients at the end of 1969. If the old pattern of the annual upward trend in the resident patient population had not been interrupted in 1955, there would be over 750,000 patients in our mental hospitals. This steady decrease in the patient population has saved over six billion dollars for patient maintenance and the cost of construction of additional facilities which would have been needed if the hospital population had continued to grow at the pre-1955 rate.

Beside the salutary decrease in the patient population, a transformation has occurred in mental hospitals in the past two decades that defies description. Visit one today. You will be impressed by the serenity you observe and feel. You will sense the attitude of realistic optimism that predominates. Flowers, curtains, paintings, music, fresh air, comfortable tidy lounges make a pleasant environment for clean, tranquil patients being offered a myriad of therapies designed to make their hospitalization profitable and not a living hell. Some modern psychiatric hospitals have an almost country-club atmosphere. All are becoming what we have always wanted—attractive, active centers of treatment, offering hope of rehabilitation and return to the community, to family and friends, after a relatively short period of effective treatment.

WHAT WE HAVE LEARNED

From what has been accomplished with the psychotropic drugs, we have learned much about them, their assets and liabilities, and, equally important, what is needed to advance the chemical conquest of psychiatric illnesses. We now know that each neuroleptic—phenothiazine, thioxanthenes, and butyrophenones—is an effective antipsychotic drug, the successful use of which depends on a variety of factors, the most important of which are the symptoms and the type of illness and its duration. Optimal therapeutic results are most likely to be achieved in patients who are tense, anxious or excited. The more impoverished the patient's affect, the less likely it is that a neuroleptic will be helpful.

Clinical experience has confirmed that when a neuroleptic is prescribed for specific target symptoms of recent origin, the greater is the prospect of a beneficial response. In schizophrenia, for example, the rapidity with which treatment is started after the onset of the psychosis immeasurably influences the therapeutic result. The effect of these drugs is much more favorable in the first few months of schizophrenia and tends to diminish the longer the schizophrenia exists, except in unusual cases. Some chronic patients are helped, notably those in whom the affective component of the illness is marked.

It is now clear that the nature of the schizophrenic reaction also is important in determining the outcome of neuroleptic therapy. The simple schizophrenic and chronic hebephrenic rarely are benefited by these compounds. Some of the most remarkable symptomatic improvements have been achieved in the hyperkinetic catatonics, especially those who have had periods of normality between their attacks of excitement or stupor and whose basic personality is intact. Equally gratifying results have been obtained in cases of paranoid schizophrenia, paraphrenia, and paranoia where the personality is well preserved.

Neuroleptics are not curative, but adequate neuroleptic therapy enables patients to conform to conventional modes of behavior, to live at home and to work in spite of the persistence of their basic affliction. Instead of becoming less introspective, patients become more spontaneous and more productive as they are freed from disabling symptoms. Consequently, many individuals, as a result of taking these drugs, have been discharged from the hospital. There are many others who have not achieved sufficient improvement to be returned to the community but who have been removed from a disturbed to a quiet ward, who have been granted ground privileges, who can participate in more of the hospital's social and therapeutic programs, and who can make temporary home visits. For these previously severely incapacitated patients, neuroleptics have been a blessing that has eased the cross of their illness, something no previous drug therapy accomplished.

Paradoxically, each neuroleptic benefits many patients refractory to all other drug therapies. This individual therapeutic responsiveness to a particular neuroleptic suggests that genetic factors governing absorption and metabolism are very important. There is an urgent need for more research in pharmacogenetics. Such research combined with more in-depth studies of the structure-activity relationship of psychopharmaceuticals should provide us with more precise knowledge of the mode of action of these drugs and ultimately with more specific chemotherapy for emotional and mental disorders.

Equally important in determining therapeutic outcome is the administration of doses titrated to the needs of the individual. A hallmark of many neuroleptics is their extraordinary effective dosage range. This is extremely important for schizophrenics, especially the chronically ill. They often require doses far in excess of those needed by acute schizophrenics and nonschizophrenics. This suggests that chronic schizophrenics are metabolically different and because of this need and tolerate very high doses of neuroleptics. Can you imagine treating anyone but a chronic schizophrenic with 1,500 mg daily of fluphenazine?

Because of its physiologic and pharmacologic actions, each neuroleptic causes side effects of varying intensity in all patients. Yet schizophrenics, especially chronic schizophrenics, have fewer severe side effects than nonschizophrenics. They are as prone to allergic and toxic reactions, such as dermatological, hematological and hepatic reactions, as anyone else exposed to these drugs. They also are no more susceptible to extrapyramidal reactions, which are the most frequent neurophysiologic effects of the more potent neuroleptics. In fact, the overall incidence of serious side reactions to these drugs is very low among schizophrenics, in view of the millions who have received not one but several neuroleptics alone or in combination for months and years.

There is no doubt that large numbers of psychiatric patients require indefinite neuroleptic therapy. This raises questions concerning the possible effects of long-term therapy. Can improvement be maintained? Will tolerance develop, making larger and larger doses less and less effective? Will patients become addicted and develop withdrawal symptoms? Will such essential organs as liver, bone marrow and kidneys suffer from protracted therapy? What are the risks of long-term therapy to the eyes and to the skin? If a woman on indefinite therapy becomes pregnant, what hazards are there for her and the fetus?

That improvement can be sustained is exemplified by the thousands of patients in whom this has occurred as a result of taking a neuroleptic continuously for as long as 15 years. These patients often have taken progressively lower rather than increasing doses of their medication. There is no clinical evidence of tolerance to neuroleptics, nor has there been any evidence of addiction to these drugs. They can be discontinued gradually, even after years of administration, without the development of withdrawal symptoms. To date, there is no convincing clinical or laboratory evidence that protracted neuroleptic treatment has any deleterious effects on the liver, bone marrow, or kidneys.

Since women are more susceptible to psychiatric illnesses than men, it is reasonable to assume that of the millions treated with psychotropic drugs, at least a few thousand of them received one of these drugs while pregnant. A review of the world's literature on the effects of psychoactive drugs either on mothers or fetuses discloses only a very few reports of congenital defects in children whose mothers took a neuroleptic while pregnant. What is most important is the fact that these women also consumed during their pregnancy other medications that could have been responsible for the congenital abnormalities in their offspring.

Although long-term neuroleptic therapy has been safe for the majority of patients, two hazards of it warrant mention. Some phenothiazines, especially chlorpromazine, may cause a pigmentation of light-exposed skin (face, neck, hands), a pigmentation in the sclera, and conjunctiva, and/or granular deposits in the lens and cornea, producing opacities, and, in rare instances, retinal pigmentation. The larger the dose and the longer the duration of phenothiazine administration, the greater the risk of these changes in susceptible individuals. Individual sensitivity is an important variable, since this syndrome has developed in some patients who had received considerably smaller quantities of the phenothiazine than others who still have not developed skin or eye changes. The dermatologic reaction, which evolves slowly, consists of a distinctive grey, violaceous discoloration of the skin causing some patients to have a purple-grey hue. This has been reported *only* in patients treated with chlorpromazine. The exact incidence is unknown, but it is estimated to occur in less than 0.1% of all patients treated with chlorpromazine for two years or more. At the present time, this seems to constitute no more than a cosmetic problem.

Although patients with skin pigmentation have ocular complications, very many more patients have eye but no skin changes. Eye changes have been reported not only in chlorpromazine-treated patients, but also in patients on long-term levomepromazine therapy and in patients treated with thiothixene. Thus far, eye pigmentation due to these drugs has been very infrequent and only rarely has it caused any impairment of visual acuity. These drug-induced lens and corneal opacities now seem to be irreversible.

Since 1958, there has been a steady increase of published reports of a unique neurologic complication of neuroleptic therapy—persistent dyskinesia. This consists of involuntary continuous munching and masticatory movements of the patient's jaw with protrusion of the tongue and grimaces of the lips. Associated with these facial movements may be a compulsion to walk or pace the floor. When standing, the patient may incessantly rock his body forward, backward, and side to side, or constantly shift his weight from one foot to the other. Characteristically, this syndrome usually does not appear until after the drug has been taken for at least six months by a susceptible patient. It has appeared most often in patients over 60 years of age and has been uncommon in those under 50. Those familiar with persistent dyskinesia realize that it imposes severe limitations on the patient's chances of living in the community, even if there should be a remission of psychotic symptomatology. Few families, friends or neighbors would tolerate for long witnessing the abnormal movements. Hence, patients with persistent dyskinesia may have to remain in the hospital because of a complication of the therapy designed to get them out of the hospital.

Many doctors still are not fully aware of the need for continued administration of the major tranquilizers, frequently in large doses, in order to maintain adequate remission in chronically ill mental patients. Consequently, we are witnessing a new phenomenon, the "merry-go-round" process, created by the discharges and readmissions of patients whose maintenance dosage outside the hospital is reduced to inadequate levels or even discontinued. There are many chronically ill patients in the "revolving door" group who simply will not take their medication regularly, despite all efforts to persuade them to do so. In every psychiatric hospital there are patients who could be released, if they could be relied on to take medicine as prescribed. It has been estimated that as many as twenty per cent of hospital patients fail to take their drugs consistently, despite supervision. These uncooperative individuals spit out, regurgitate, hide, and discard expensive drugs, thereby impeding their rehabilitation. These two groups of drug defectors constitute a large segment of the world's psychiatric population. They have been and are a major therapeutic challenge. Since these patients, who patently need chemotherapy, are unreliable drug takers, what has been needed for them has been a long-acting depot injectable neuroleptic. Such a preparation would remove responsibility for taking medicine from patients too ill to assume it. This would assure physicians that patients are getting their medication, and would enable them to return more patients to the community and to keep them there. The development of fluphenazine enanthate, fluphenazine decanoate, and injectable flupenthixol has made this possible.

Long-acting injectable neuroleptics represent another step forward in the treatment of certain psychiatric patients. These preparations slowly release the medication into the system, providing a duration of action from two to eight weeks. Equally important is the fact that the injectable dose is only a fraction of the oral dose of the same drug. In some instances, for example, 25 mg fluphenazine enanthate every two weeks was as effective as 700 mg oral fluphenazine in the same period of time; in others 25 mg fluphenazine enanthate every two weeks was as effective as 8,400 mg or 12,600 mg chlorpromazine orally over 14 days. Whether this unusual and unique duration of action of small doses of long-acting injectable neuroleptics is due to the rate of absorption or metabolism or a totally different mode of action is unknown at present. Because the judicious use of these preparations has kept many patients out of hospitals who in the past either would not have been released or who would have had repeated readmissions, I predict that more long-acting injectable neuroleptics will be developed and that this form of treatment will be used more extensively.

Although I have stressed the safety of and necessity for prolonged neuroleptic therapy, it also is true that intermittent neuroleptic therapy or "drug holidays" are feasible for many patients because a characteristic of these drugs is their ability to bind to body tissues from which they are released slowly after the medication is stopped. The number of chronically ill patients in and out of hospitals who are receiving continuous drug therapy that they may not need is unknown. There is reason to believe that 25% to 30% could benefit from drug holidays for a minimum of eight to 12 weeks, that 75% could be without drug for 3 to 4 weeks, and that 90% or more could be maintained on drug holidays of one to 14 days.

In view of the accumulated clinical evidence that intermittent chemotherapy is feasible for selected chronically ill psychiatric patients without increasing morbidity, psychiatrists should consider a program of drug holidays for these individuals. Such a program offers many advantages. The possible risk of toxic effects from a continuous chemical assault on the body would be lessened. The hazard of the recently recognized complications of long-term, continuous neuroleptic therapy, such as skin and eye changes and persistent dyskinesia, may be minimized by drug holidays.

It is often said that all neuroleptics, minor tranquilizers, and antidepressants are essentially the same and that there are no major differences between them. This is misleading and quite deceptive. There are important differences between these drugs, related, in part, to the differences in chemical structure. The latter profoundly influences the milligram potency, the duration of action, and the type and frequency of side effects. The variety of psychoactive drugs available makes it possible to select a specific drug most likely to benefit the individual patient with the least risk.

In the past decade drug abuse has become a major public health problem. Yet, despite the fact that psychoactive drugs have been prescribed for millions of patients, including individuals prone to drug abuse, there is no evidence of substantial abuse of these drugs. Abuse of neuroleptics and the antidepressants has not been recorded. Only certain minor tranquilizers have been accused of being abused drugs. These are the ones that have proven clinically the most effective and the most widely dispensed of all the minor tranquilizers.

The actual frequency of abuse of minor tranquilizers encountered in medical practice is very difficult to determine. There is a minimum of reports in the world's medical literature suggesting that minor tranquilizers have been abused by a very small number of individuals. An analysis of these discloses that the patients almost always were psychopathic personalities with histories of abuse of alcohol or drugs, most often barbiturates or nonbarbiturate hypnotics, which they had obtained from legitimate sources. Rarely, if ever, did these patients abuse a single drug. On the contrary, they invariably consumed two or more drugs, often with large quantities of alcohol. Typically, they self-medicated with these combinations of minor tranquilizers, sedatives and alcohol for anxiety, depression, vaguely described "nervousness," and/or insomnia. In most instances, psychic dependence on these combinations preceded a physical dependence, if the latter occurred.

An evaluation of the available data on abusers of minor tranquilizers compels these conclusions:

1/ The potential for abuse of these drugs, like the potential for abuse of any pharmaceutical, does occur.

2/ The number of abusers in the world constitutes an insignificantly small percentage of the millions who have been exposed to the minor tranquilizers. The percentage is so small it can hardly be calculated.

3/ The abuse of these drugs is a reflection of the psychopathology of the user rather than a manifestation of something inherent in the drugs themselves.

4/ There is no evidence that a serious problem has been created for society by the infinitesimally few abusers of these compounds.

The existence of abusers of minor tranquilizers raises some questions that command serious thought. Why do they self-medicate, that is, use drugs obtained legitimately in doses above those recommended by the prescribing physician? Is it possible that the doctor underestimated the dosage required by the patient to obtain the symptomatic relief sought? Why is it that so-called abusers seldom, if ever, continuously raise the dose taken but stop at the level that suffices for their needs? Is this real abuse or does it represent either an effort on the part of the individual to secure surcease from subjective discomfort or the pathologic seeking of a peculiar state of mind through drugs? Some alleged abusers not only immediately cease this when a more effective drug is prescribed but they take the new medication as recommended. This suggests that their abuse of the prior medication was an effort on their part to achieve symptomatic relief and not a drug-induced pathologic psychic state. Hence, some abuse of minor tranquilizers can be attributed to the inept choice of medication by the prescribing physician or a problem that exists because the medical profession lacks drugs suitable for the legitimate needs of some distressed people.

Although vast quantities of minor tranquilizers have been prescribed, it must be stated that not all have been dispensed judiciously by some practitioners. Such misuse is indicative of physicians who unwisely accede to the demands of patients or who supplant sound clinical judgment for expediency. The disregard of these doctors for the potential abuse of minor tranquilizers and for the welfare of their patients is further manifested by their prescribing large quantities with no restrictions on refills and with no insistence that the patient return at regular intervals for evaluation of the response to or the need for the medication. It also is true that far too often many pharmacists supply patients with these drugs without ascertaining if they are still under a physician's care. These practices not only warrant condemnation but invite drug abuse. Clearly, the abuse of some psychoactive drugs may call for the indictment of physicians and pharmacists rather than the drugs.

PRESENT AND FUTURE NEEDS

There are those who think there are too many psychotropic drugs. These individuals fail to recognize that none of the available compounds are universally effective and safe. They overlook the indisputable fact that, despite all the psychoactive drugs on hand, there are in and outside of mental hospitals many thousands of patients either partially or totally refractory to these drugs or intolerant of them. For these unfortunate, suffering individuals, there is an urgent need for more psychotropic drugs. Those who would limit the number of psychotropic drugs also ignore what every psychiatrist experienced in testing and using these drugs knows, namely, that some patients benefit only from one compound and are unresponsive to, or are intolerant of, all other drugs. Thus, for those patients who respond to a particular tranquilizer or antidepressant, old or new, that one drug is invaluable; it means for them the difference between sickness and health even if, in comparison to all other drugs, it would seem to be the least effective. This is most important for these patients because humans and not statistics suffer. The challenge to the medical profession comes not from the number of drugs available, but from the need to learn the art of using these drugs correctly. The simple clinical fact is that the more drugs we have at our disposal, the greater is the number of patients who will be helped.

The foundations for the salutary achievements of biological psychiatry were laid by our numerous predecessors who, although principally clinicans concerned with diagnosis and treatment, demonstrated that the brain is not simply an electrical or computer-like mechanism but a complex chemical system as well. With enviable and exemplary dedication and skill, these pioneers worked with patients whose illnesses were refractory to all therapeutic intervention. Their persistence and their willingness to take legitimate risks resulted in the important scientific advances and therapeutic triumphs of biological psychiatry we now acclaim.

Biological psychiatry is partially the product of cross-fertilization of ideas. The research-minded psychiatrist no longer can rely exclusively on his own efforts. He must depend also not alone on the independent contributions of workers in a number of related disciplines but on an interchange with them. This is why biological psychiatrists already work with physiologists, pharmacologists, biochemists, geneticists, bioengineers, statisticians, psychologists, social scientists and others. We are accustomed to transdisciplinary teamwork at many levels. There must be more of this for further progress to be made.

One major obstacle to the advancement of chemopsychiatry is the contemporary paucity of clinical psychiatrists who labor to improve their diagnostic competence, their therapeutic skills, and the astuteness and scientific validity of their clinical observations. Biological psychiatry needs clinicians who also strive to become more of a scientist familiar with all the tools employed by the modern scientist. Biological psychiatry has made it more relevant and more imperative for the psychiatrist to study neuroanatomy, neurophysiology, neuronendocrinology, neurochemistry, pharmacology, genetics, ethology, and medical statistics as well as psychology, learning theory, sociology, anthropology, demography and epidemiology.

While we wait for research to produce safer and more universally effective psychotropic drugs, I am convinced that much more can be accomplished with the available psychopharmaceuticals. Clinicians could learn more about pharmacogenetics and about the nature of psychiatric illnesses and their treatment with the medicines we have by making more astute clinical observations, by more experimentation with wider dosage ranges, and by careful trials of combined psychotropic drug therapy. In my opinion, many more patients could attain more optimal therapeutic results with the available psychotropics if more physicians paid more attention to individual susceptibility to a drug. The sad truth is that not enough doctors have mastered the art of psychopharmacotherapy, and that this accounts for the divergent therapeutic results and complications reported by different therapists. It is an indictment of physicians that we have not accomplished all that could be achieved in the treatment of psychiatric patients with the available psychotropic drugs.

EPILOGUE

When medical historians name the chief advances in the second half of the twentieth century, organ transplantation and nucleic acid chemistry will rank high, but it may be that the increased understanding of pharmacological events underlying human physiology, disease, and behavior will be given an even higher place. For it is from this progress that a more rational approach to the production of specific therapeutic agents may develop.

As we contemplate what biological psychiatry has accomplished, it is imperative that we realize the immense power we now possess to intervene in the nonintellectual functions of the brain and to alter moods and emotional states. It is clear that chemicals affect the functioning of the brain and that we now are able to influence the brain in ways heretofore impossible. As the chemistry of the brain is more definitively known and a growing range of drugs that affect its functions is synthesized, an increasingly extensive and precise influence over how a person thinks, feels and behaves surely will be possible. Biological psychiatry already is an important part of the growing technology for controlling human behavior. To some this is cause for cheering, but to others the future is fraught with terrors for man. The latter need not be if we aspire to moral grandeur, and if we face the ethical problems posed by scientific and technological developments. Science will forge ahead because each discovery inspires more research and development. If we labor as assiduously to develop our inner spiritual wealth as we have labored to maximize our material, physical and mental well-being, the future is full of hope for man. Whether we shall be praised or cursed by our children's children will depend on how much we succeed today in being aware of the value of human life and of our extensive obligation to the individual and to society.

Index of Subjects